# The Acquisition
## of Motor Skill

Matthew Kleinman

Brooklyn College of the
City University of New York

PRINCETON BOOK COMPANY, *Publishers*
PRINCETON NEW JERSEY

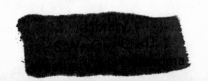

To Joan, Jon, and Liza

The illustrations in this text have been reproduced with permission from the publishers:

Figure 4-1 from *The Transfer of Learning* by Henry Ellis (Macmillan Publishing Co., Inc., Copyright © 1965 by Henry Ellis); Figure 4-2 from *The Psychology of Learning* (2nd ed.) by James Deese (McGraw-Hill Book Co., Inc., Copyright © 1958); Figures 6-2, 6-5, 6-6, 6-10 from *Human Physiology* (2nd ed.) by Arthur J. Vander, James H. Sherman, and Dorothy S. Luciano (McGraw-Hill Book Co., Inc., Copyright © 1970, 1975); Figure 6-3 from *Functional Human Anatomy* (2nd ed.) by James E. Crouch (Lea & Febiger, Copyright © 1972); Figure 6-4 from *Bionics* edited by Ryszard Gawronski (Elsevier-North Holland Publishing Co., Copyright © 1971); Figures 6-7, 6-11, 6-12 from *Physiology of the Nervous System* (2nd ed.) by Carlos Eyzaguirre and Salvatore J. Fidone (Year Book Medical Publishers, Inc., Copyright © 1969, 1975); Figure 6-8 from *The Neurosciences: Third Study Program* edited by Francis O. Schmitt and Frederic G. Worden (The MIT Press, Copyright © 1974); Figure 6-9 from *Readings in Neurophysiology* by Charles D. Barnes and Christopher Kircher (John Wiley & Sons, Inc., Copyright © 1968)

Library of Congress Catalog Card Number 81-84597
ISBN 0-916622-24-X
Printed in the United States of America

# Table of Contents

# Introduction

MOVEMENT IS A CRITICAL FACTOR in human learning; not only does it provide a means of physical and emotional expression, but it is often indicative of the presence of life itself. It serves as the vehicle for the translation of thought into action and constitutes the mechanism through which the organism can interact with its environment. The acquisition of motor skills is essential to the growth and development of the individual and serves as a rewarding experience in its own right.

The purpose of this book is to provide the reader with factual information and with insight into the theoretical, methodological, and physiological factors essential to understanding the fundamental processes which underlie the acquisition of motor skills. The theoretical foundations of motor learning are viewed within their historical context and are traced to such diverse disciplines as philosophy, neurophysiology, psychology, and physical education. While there is much in this book that will reinforce educational practices that have been adopted intuitively, it is hoped that by increasing the reader's awareness of the underlying theoretical factors, methods employed in teaching and coaching can be refined and made more effective. It is also a major intention of this work to enlighten physical educators to the undesirable nature of certain teaching procedures which have been adopted in the absence of either experimental evidence or theoretical justification.

This book is organized into two major sections: the first deals with theoretical and methodological considerations; the second is concerned with the learner as a processor of information. The first section describes the evolution and development of the major theoretical controversies which have dominated motor learning research for the first half of this century. Since motor learning theories are predicated largely upon experimental findings, it is felt that the reader should be provided with basic concepts concerning the inherent limitations of those statistical methods most commonly employed in motor learning research, thus increasing comprehension and critical evaluation of the research literature. Such heightened insight into the interpretation and application of research findings should ultimately result in the formulation of more effective teaching practices.

Particular emphasis has been placed upon the areas of transfer of learning and practice distribution—historically significant and widely researched—which are fundamental to the study of such contemporary issues as the effects of knowledge of results upon the acquisition of skill and the role of motor memory in its retention. How transfer of learning and practice distribution affect motor skill acquisition is studied from a dual perspective: the capacity of the learner and the taxonomy (nature) of the criterion task. Since differences in these factors exert a critical effect upon the outcome of an experimental study, they must always be considered when evaluating research findings in learning transfer and practice distribution. This section of the book attempts to clarify the role of transfer in motor learning and to eliminate common misconceptions about its nature. The effects of practice distribution are discussed in relation to the planning and scheduling of instructional programs.

The examination of the neurophysiological mechanisms in motor behavior focuses upon the functional role of the nervous system in the learning and control of movement, rather than on its structural aspects. In order to accomplish this end, anatomical and physiological detail has been subordinated to the overriding concept of the nervous system as an information-processing mechanism. While particular neurological structures are described, their functions are discussed in the light of research on their role in the mediation of motor behavior. The primary objective of this section of the book, then, is to provide the reader with insight concerning the integrative action of the nervous system in the mediation of complex, goal-directed motor activity.

Differences in neurological functioning result in differences in an individual's capacity to process information. The second section of the text deals with the learner as an active participant in the acquisition process. Some individuals are skilled at verbal activities; others tend to perform better upon motor tasks. The extent to which these abilities affect the capacity to learn is a matter of interest to teachers and coaches alike. A major source of controversy is whether abilities are innate factors which are genetically determined, or whether they constitute behavioral traits modified by experience. The role of individual differences in motor learning is examined from the standpoint of the need to interface the abilities of the learner with the requirements of the task.

The advent of the computer has given rise to a body of theory related to the systematic processing of information. Current views concerning the nature of motor learning are based upon the application of this information theory to skill acquisition. These theoretical models are, in turn, based upon the structure and function of the nervous system and place great stress upon the role of feedback in the learning process. Knowledge of results is a type of feedback valuable in facilitating skill acquisition. The text provides guidelines, based upon current research, for the most effective applications of knowledge of results to teaching skills. Both closed- and open-loop theoretical models of learning are discussed, taking into account their implications in the acquisition and performance of motor activities.

Motor learning is dependent upon a precise knowledge of what is to be done and an awareness of the means through which a given goal can be accomplished. The learning and performance of motor skills is contingent upon the learner's capacity to process verbal, visual, and kinesthetic information through cognitive and spatial frames of reference. These reference mechanisms are formed through reinforced practice. If it is not properly reinforced by knowledge of results, practice will result in frustration and the adoption of haphazard, trial-and-error methods which will worsen rather than heighten performance. This book is predicated upon the belief that motor learning is best facilitated by instructional methods based upon theoretical and experimental evidence. While some of the intuitively adopted methods traditionally employed in the teaching of motor skills are valid, others are not. The analysis and discussion of factual information within the appropriate theoretical context will enable the teacher of motor skills to evaluate current methods more effectively and will provide, as well, the critical insight for the development of new ones.

# PART I

## Theory and Method

# CHAPTER 1

# Motor Learning in Historical Perspective

HUMAN MOVEMENT IS DECEPTIVE in its overt simplicity. To the casual observer, the ease with which the dancer leaps, the precision of the skilled athlete, the grace of the gymnast all represent physical acts which appear to have little or no relationship to learned behavior. Actually, the acquisition of motor skills is a complex process which entails the interaction between physiological and behavioral factors. Motor learning results in the acquisition of complex, goal-directed activities which are ultimately executed in a manner that is indistinguishable from that which governs innate reflexive responses. A major objective of motor learning research is to provide insight into the mechanisms which underlie the acquisition and performance of complex, purposive motor activities.

The fundamental concepts governing the acquisition and performance of motor skills are rooted in philosophical issues. The nature-nurture controversy (environment versus heredity) and the mind-body dichotomy (the mental versus the physical), for example, provide the philosophical framework for a number of the contemporary issues involved in the study of motor learning. Twentieth-century advances in knowledge about the structure and function of the nervous system can facilitate the understanding of skill acquisition only when such information is analyzed within the appropriate theoretical context. Although experimental methodology is a powerful tool of scientific research, it must be realized that the initial design and the ultimate interpretation of the findings of an experiment are critically dependent upon theoretical guidelines which are themselves based upon fundamental philosophical concepts.

Many of the methods and practices currently employed in teaching motor skills are intuitive approaches which have been developed in the absence of appropriate theoretical justification. While such methods may prove adequate under a given set of conditions, they may fail totally if any of the parameters of the learning situation—e.g., the age and sex of the subjects, the nature of the criterion task, or the temporal distribution of work and rest—are altered. It is hoped that just as in the physical sciences the work of Isaac Newton clarified and systematized information which had been intuitively obvious for centuries, advances in the biological and behavioral sciences can provide a rigorous framework for the study of motor skill acquisition. In order to accomplish this end, however, it is necessary to develop a language powerful enough to relate the factors which determine the structure and function of an organism to those which govern its interaction with the environment.

In the broadest sense, this dynamic interaction between organism and environment constitutes behavior. Learning may be defined as a long-term change in behavior which results from the effects of practice. To understand the nature of motor learning, identification of those factors which interact with the functioning of the organism and elicit predictable, long-lasting behavioral changes is needed. Great care in the pursuit of these ends is advised, because there are a number of factors other than learned responses that can exert long-term behavioral effects. Maturation, for example, is a major competitor to learning in eliciting behavioral change. Maturational changes occur solely as a function of time, while learned behavior is the direct result of practice. The study of motor skill acquisition is particularly confounded during childhood and adolescence when it is exceedingly difficult to separate the effects of learning from those of maturation.

The factors which affect skill acquisition may be divided into three broad categories:

1.  Those related to the nature and conditions of the learning situation, such as the temporal distribution of practice (the relative frequency of work and rest), the serial order of instruction, or the nature and frequency of reinforcement.

2.  Those which pertain to the nature of the learner, such as individual differences in age, sex, motivation, and ability level.

3.  Those which relate to the taxonomy of the learning task, such as speed, pacing, complexity, and coherence.

Since motor learning is dependent upon the dynamic interaction between the learner and the environment, it is necessary to formulate clear relationships between the effects of given environmental manipulations and the capacity of the learner to acquire specific skills. The understanding of the fundamental nature of these dynamic processes will be greatly facilitated once such lawful relationships have been established. For example, how will the temporal distribution of practice interact with the learner's capacity to process information? Will the magnitude of these interactions vary with the age and sex of the learner? Will the effects of practice distribution vary with taxonomical differences in the learning task? Will high-ability subjects perform better under a given temporal distribution of practice than those of low ability? How will the serial order in which skills are taught interact with the learner's capacity for retention and recall? Under the same conditions, will transfer of learning be proportionately greater for high-ability than for low-ability individuals? How will the taxonomical factors of the learning task affect transfer?

Clearly, these are complex issues which can only be resolved through a concerted research effort. Such an effort can be strongly influenced, however, by intuitive knowledge and practical experience. For example, the performance of students practicing under conditions which are reinforced by knowledge of results (a form of extrinsic verbal feedback) is consistently superior to that of students of equal ability practicing under trial-and-error conditions. Individuals practicing under distributed conditions (periods of work separated by periods of rest) generally outperform those working under massed practice (continuous practice with no rest). Students who are taught to perform a given criterion task from the outset of training tend ultimately to outperform those intially trained on a similar, yet distinct, "lead-up" activity prior to learning the criterion task. A major objective of motor learning research entails the identification and explanation of the theoretical principles which underlie these readily observable phenomena.

Given the advances in knowledge of the structure and function of the nervous system, the application of information-processing models to skill acquisition research constitutes one of the more productive theoretical approaches. Proponents of information theory are far from unanimity in their respective views of the precise elements critical to learning. There are two fundamentally opposing groups, centralists and peripheralists, among those favoring information-processing models of motor control. Centralists hypothesize an outflow model and argue the primacy of predetermined motor programs which are stored in memory and selectively called out in the initiation and control of specific movements. The centralists contend that the pattern of impulses transmitted from the motor area of the brain to the involved muscles during an evolving movement is accompanied by a corollary discharge or efference copy which ultimately gives rise to the conscious perception of movement. The peripheralists, in contrast, advocate an inflow model of motor control in which the evolving movement is continually adjusted and refined in the light of information feedback generated by specialized receptors in the muscles, joints, and tendons of the involved limb segments. The peripheralists argue that it is this information feedback which gives rise to the conscious perception of movement. While inflow and outflow models appear antithetical, current research indicates that motor learning entails both central and peripheral processes, and that the respective importance of each varies with the nature of the learning task. A productive approach to the study of motor learning must account for the interactions between the nature of the learning task and the information-processing capacity of the learner.

The earliest inquiries into the nature of learning were carried out within the discipline of philosophy. Such concepts as contiguity (learning through association) and reflex action were initially subsumed in the broad context of formal philosophical argument, but were ultimately clarified and defined through scientific and technological advances in the biological sciences, particularly physiology. The synthesis of knowledge derived from philosophy and physiology became a precursor to the evolution of the behavioral science of psychology. Philosophy and physiology gave rise to many of the fundamental issues associated with motor learning, but it was the discipline of psychology that provided a language for discussing them in purely behavioral terms. Although such behavioral language has clarified and defined certain basic issues, they remain far from resolved. The plethora of definitions of learning is unfortunately accompanied by a paucity of knowledge pertaining to its essential nature. The literature abounds with theories of motor learning, but the mechanisms which govern the translation of thought into action remain largely undiscovered. Although many of the basic issues are unresolved, current theoretical and experimental research conducted within the area of physical education has significantly furthered knowledge of the nature of motor learning.

### Philosophical Influences

The historical background of motor learning is thus complex and varied. Motor learning is largely concerned with the processes which underlie the acquisition of motor skills, and no single individual may rightfully be identified as the founder of the field. Its philosophical foundations can be traced to the rational philosophy of René Descartes and the empiricism of John Locke, George Berkeley, and David Hume.

Descartes envisioned the human body as a machine whose function could be explained through the application of the principles of physics. He was aware that movement resulted from the coordinated action of opposing pairs of muscles and realized that the nervous system constituted the physical basis for both sensation and movement. In his "pathway" theory of the peripheral nervous system, Descartes initiated the modern concept of the reflex arc, a critical factor in the processes which underlie the acquisition of motor skills. Although fundamentally dualistic in nature, his distinction between mind and body gave rise to the contemporary position dichotomizing motoric and ideational activities. Descartes was also among the first to hypothesize the brain as the locus of thought, reason, and volitional activity; by so doing, he gave rise to the interactionist approach to the study of human behavior which characterizes much of contemporary learning research. Descartes was concerned with the physical mechanisms governing the workings of the body itself and believed that capacities for thought and reason constituted mere factors which were innate functions of its organization. An individual could think, learn, and reason because there were physical mechanisms within the body which are programed to execute these functions. Locke, however, took great exception to the idea of innate capacities for the processes of learning and thinking, contending instead that the ultimate source of all knowledge is experience.

These fundamental theoretical differences have given rise to the nature-nurture controversy, which concerns itself with the respective roles of heredity and environmental factors in learning and performance. Advocates of heredity as the major factor in determining an individual's capacity for a given activity argue that human abilities are largely predetermined by biological factors and that experience plays only a minimal role in the level of achievement an individual attains. This view of human development is known as determinism, and while there are a few outspoken contemporary advocates of this position, it currently enjoys little popular acceptance. In contrast to the determinists' view, proponents of environmental and cultural influences upon human development contend that the central element in learning is not biological but experiential. The old adage, champions are made and not born, is a classical example of the environmentalist position. The behaviorists are the leading contemporary advocates of the central role of environmental factors in learning, arguing that an individual is the product of his environment rather than his heredity. The individual is viewed as a blank slate, and it is solely the experiences of life that determine what will ultimately be inscribed.

Locke was among the first to purport that sensation arising from physical experience is essential to the formulation of ideas. Arguing that experience sets the limits of knowledge, he contended that although an individual is capable of abstract reasoning, all ideas must be ultimately reducible to sensory input. Locke also differentiated between simple and complex behavior, arguing that the basic element of even the simplest idea must constitute some form of sensory experience, such as the perception of color, odor, or texture. Complex ideas evolve from abstractions drawn from the interactions occuring among the simple ideas. Locke's premise regarding the primacy of sensory experience in the evolution of complex ideational activities has been adopted by contemporary theorists in the area of child development (Jean Piaget

[1968] is a leading proponent of this position), who assert that motor activity constitutes one of the most essential primary elements in the development of thought and reason.

Locke's contention that there could be no thought in the absence of experience and sensation was adopted by Berkeley, who placed particular emphasis upon the role of visual sensation in the processes governing thought and learning. Berkeley modified the prevailing contemporary theory of visual perception to include tactile mediation (touch), as well as visual and kinesthetic cues. This modification was based upon his argument that the formulation of spatial concepts, such as width and depth, develops only through the association of visual, kinesthetic, and tactile sensations within the context of an actual experience. He wholly rejected the idea of abstraction, arguing that at best one can only isolate the components of particular ideas. Time and space, for example, cannot exist outside of a specific situation in which they can be completely measured.

While the findings of contemporary physics have clearly dispelled Berkeley's arguments regarding time and space, his general ideas concerning abstraction have particular relevance to some of the current issues within motor learning. Since a motor skill is a highly specific entity requiring the exertion of muscular force within precise temporal and spatial limits, the quest to abstract the factors of general motor ability which underlie successful motor performance has thus far failed to yield any substantive findings. No matter how similar two motor skills may appear, each is unique in terms of its temporal and spatial patterning. The forehand stroke in tennis and badminton, for example, may appear overtly similar but involve very different patterns of muscular force and timing.

Of all the empirical philosophers, it is the work of Hume which has made the greatest single contribution to the development of contemporary learning theory. Hume expanded Locke's distinction between simple and complex ideas by further differentiating ideas from sensations. Just as there exist both simple and complex ideas, there are also simple and complex sensations. While an idea (goodness, happiness, intelligence) can exist independently of physical experience, a sensation is the direct result of some form of concrete activity. An experienced tennis player can tell when a ball is well hit solely from the "feel" of its contact with the racket. Hume argued that abstract reasoning processes are valuable in such theoretical activities as formal logic and the derivation of mathematical propositions, but have little value when dealing with concrete matters of fact. Hume's differentiation between abstract and concrete processes gave rise to the distinction between the motoric and the ideational aspects of motor learning. The abstract or nonspecific aspects of motor skill acquisition pertain to the rules and principles which govern the conduct of the activity, while the specific or motoric aspects pertain to those temporal and spatial factors governing the precise execution of muscular force.

Perhaps Hume's most salient contribution to the development of modern learning theory is his principle of cause and effect. The cause of any event must always precede its effect and, conversely, the effect must always follow the cause. In order for a given stimulus to be considered the cause of a particular response (effect), that stimulus, when present, must always result in the occurrence of that response, and, conversely, the response will occur only when preceded by the particular stimulus (cause). A professional baseball player will bunt only when given the signal to do so. Should the player manifest a response other than bunting, he will be subject to a fine or suspension. Conversely, a player will not bunt unless so instructed. In this example, the coach's signal is the cause and the player's response (bunting) is the effect. In a cause and effect relationship, the effect can be explained in terms of the presence of the causal element. Association is dependent upon the proximity of the occurrence of both events. The critical element governing the association between a cause and an effect is the close temporal contiguity (proximity) in which the events occur. If a sizeable time interval exists between the occurrence of the respective events, association will not take place. Hume's principle of contiguity has been adopted as the fundamental theoretical element governing the phenomenon of classical conditioning, and many contemporary learning theorists, particularly in the area of child development, contend that contiguity constitutes the basic element of all learning.

There are many practical examples of contiguous association in the realm of human learning. An infant learns to associate the physiological satisfaction derived from the formula contained in his bottle with the sight and feel of the bottle itself. In a game of baseball, the signals the catcher gives to the pitcher are perceived as meaningless by the spectators, yet each gesture has in fact been contiguously associated with a specific command for a given pitch. It is even argued by some theorists that language itself is basically a process of contiguous association between given objects or events and particular patterns of sound.

The empiricism of Locke, Berkeley, and Hume was often rejected on the grounds that it was simply too naive to provide a satisfactory explanation for the complex processes involved in learning, thinking, and reasoning. Immanuel Kant theorized that learning must entail some inherent capacity for codifying and organizing sensory input. He felt that although experience is essential, the most critical factor in learning is the limits of the learner's capacity to process sensory input in an efficient and systematic manner. The current concepts of basic motor abilities are rooted in Kant's philosophical principles which regard abilities as organismic capacities for processing specific types of information. While a group of individuals may be exposed to identical methods of instruction, there will be clear differences among its members in the rates of learning and levels of proficiency attained. The origin of these differences—factors which are innate, acquired through experience, or the result of the interaction between the environment and heredity—is currently the subject of much heated philosophical debate and intensive scientific investigation.

A current source of such controversy exists between behavioristic learning theorists and cognitive theorists, the argument centering on the role of organizational factors in learning. Behaviorists contend that learning results from contiguous association or reinforcement following a series of attempts based solely upon trial and error. Cognitive theorists argue that learning is the result of insight and problem-solving activities, both of which are critically dependent upon capacities (cognitive structures) for ordering and organizing information. They say that neither association nor reinforcement can account for the processes underlying complex forms of human learning, since learning results *not* from the random association of external events through trial and error, but from a capacity within the individual to organize and interpret information.

Much of the current research in motor learning is reductionist oriented. The proponents of this philosophical position contend that it is necessary to reduce a body of data to the most fundamental and theoretical level in order to subject it to meaningful interpretation. The prominent issues in motor learning, for example, are often discussed in the language of behavioral science, which purportedly allows the problem under investigation to be analyzed within a broad theoretical context. Behavioral issues are themselves reducible to the "higher language" of the more fundamental discipline of neurophysiology, which is further reducible to even more fundamental levels, such as biochemistry, biophysics, and biomathematics. Opponents of reductionism contend that given properties exist at particular levels of organization and that these properties are lost when the discussion of the phenomena under investigation is reduced to a more fundamental level. One cannot, for example, convey adequately the properties of a hot, freshly baked apple pie by discussing the fundamental properties of each of the individual ingredients that go into it.

The structuralists, who are among the leading opponents of reductionism, contend that behavior is a complex entity in and of itself and cannot be meaningfully reduced to physiological terms. Since behavioral entities can be discussed only in the language of behavior, complex activities cannot be reduced adequately to a series of underlying physical functions. The motor skills taught within the context of physical education programs, for example, constitute highly complex behavioral entities which are themselves comprised of more fundamental physiological components. Although the acquisition of basic gymnastic skills is contingent upon the presence of such physiological abilities as strength, endurance, and flexibility, proficiency in gymnastics can be assessed only in terms of performance upon the skills themselves. A knowledge of a subject's abilities prior to learning can provide insight into his propensity for acquiring specific skills, but such measures are essentially valueless in the assessment of proficiency in a particular skill area.

Structuralists contend that there are fundamental processes of the mind which govern all forms of learning, and it is therefore possible to account for all behavior through basic general laws which govern these processes. Clearly, structuralism did not provide the appropriate philosophical climate for the evolution of motor learning. It was the advent of functionalism which ultimately provided the philosophical milieu conducive to the development of motor learning as an identifiable area of behavioral research.

Functionalism is rooted in the belief that behavior constitutes a dynamic interaction entailing ideational, motoric, and physiological factors between the organism and its environment. Perhaps the greatest single contribution of functionalism lies in its recognition of the specificity of learning and its resultant distinction between motoric and ideational activities. Functionalists were among the first to realize that the nature of the learning task, the initial state of the learner, and the specific conditions of practice all constitute critically important factors in the learning process. The gross distinction between verbal and motoric activities was further refined to distinguish rote from complex verbal learning and gross motor activities from fine ones. Functionalists recognized the critical role of the conditions of practice in the learning process, and they were particularly concerned with the effects of the length and distribution of the practice period and the effects of prior experience upon learning. Among their more significant contributions have been the recognition of the existence of individual differences and the realization that such differences are the result of biological as well as environmental factors.

Above all, functionalism was not bound by any body of universal principles, but was guided instead by an eclectic approach to specific problems in the area of behavior and learning. Although aware of the shortcomings of reductionism, functionalists were not averse to applying reductionist principles to a behavioral problem if it were believed that such an approach could provide the most satisfactory solution. It is due precisely to the functionalist reliance upon reductionist principles that the study of neurophysiology has become a matter of prime importance for many contemporary investigators in the area of human learning.

### The Neurophysiological-Neuroanatomical Background

Ideas initiated within the realm of pure philosophical speculation, such as those of Descartes, ultimately provided a theoretical framework for experimental research on the relationships of the structure and function of the nervous system to the regulation and control of movement. Philosophical issues concerning the role of sensory feedback and the inherent capacity of the learner to process information in an organized and systematic fashion gave rise to the search for the anatomical locus of specialized sensory receptors and the specific pathways through which the information they generate is conveyed to higher centers within the nervous system. Although such experimental research in neuroanatomy and neurophysiology has greatly enhanced our understanding of the role of the nervous system in the learning and performance of motor skills, the knowledge gleaned from these areas must be viewed within a unifying theoretical context if it is to be given form and definition. Since the ultimate nature of any theoretical frame of reference is philosophical, the values and precepts which guide the researcher exert a critical effect on his or her interpretation of the findings.

For centuries the study of human physical functioning and behavior was dominated by such metaphysical concepts as mechanism and vitalism. Although the existence of motor and sensory nerves was first hypothesized by the ancient Roman physician, Galen, these structures were believed to constitute a mere passive vehicle for the conduction of the animal spirits. The concept of reflex activity originally pertained to the reflection of the vital spirits from the nerves to the muscles, and it was not until the early nineteenth century that Charles Bell and François Magendie, working independently of one another, discovered the actual physiological basis of sensory and motor functions.

Bell clearly demonstrated that the dorsal roots of the spinal cord contain sensory fibers only, while the ventral portion contains the motor fibers. (See Figure 6-3 for a diagrammatic representation of the spinal cord and accompanying discussion of its functional organization.) In addition, he postulated the presence of the sensory and motor tracts within the cord, as well as the existence of distinct sensory and motor areas within the brain itself. By far, Bell's most significant contribution to the understanding of the basis of motor control lies in his concept of a kinesthetic sense arising from the muscle itself. He put forth the first cybernetic theory of motor control in his example of the "nervous circle"—kinesthetic feedback information from the active muscle critically aids in the regulation and control of motor activity. Bell also initiated the concept of the reciprocal innervation of antagonistic muscles, and, although he failed to identify the phenomenon of inhibition, he paved the way for the understanding of the fundamental mechanisms governing posture and locomotion.

The physical basis of motor control was further clarified through research on the neurophysiology of the gross phenomenon of reflex action. In 1751, Robert Whytt demonstrated that physical stimulation could produce movement in a frog even though the connection between its brain and spinal cord had been severed. Whytt directly linked reflex activity to the spinal cord and distinguished between voluntary movements, which result from a conscious or willful act, and involuntary movements, which occur in the absence of conscious mediation. Whytt's most salient contribution to the area of motor learning, however, lies in his recognition of the interaction of conscious and unconscious factors in the regulation and control of motor activities. He argued that, in the case of activities such as walking, the movement is consciously initiated but reflexively regulated.

In spite of Whytt's findings, much controversy and confusion persisted over the clear distinction between voluntary and involuntary activity. More than eighty years after Whytt had published his initial findings, Marshall Hall attempted to clarify the issues pertaining to the factors governing conscious and unconscious movement. Hall distinguished four kinds of bodily movements: 1) those consciously initiated by the cerebral cortex; 2) movements of the intercostal muscles and the diaphragm in respiration under the control of the medulla; 3) involuntary movement resulting from the contractile properties of muscle in response to direct mechanical or electrical stimulation; and 4) reflex movement, which was wholly dependent upon the spinal cord and independent of the conscious control of the brain.

Hall's position generated much controversy, particularly concerning the problem of integrating conscious processes and reflex activities. The study of the integration of voluntary and involuntary activities has exerted a strong influence upon the area of motor learning; many of the currently accepted learning theories are based upon the conditioning of reflexive responses to environmental stimuli. Although there had been much speculation about the role of reflexes in the regulation and control of behavior, it remained to the Russian physiologist, I. M. Sechenov, to provide empirical evidence which conclusively demonstrated that peripheral reflexes could be inhibited by a central cortical mechanism. Sechenov formalized these findings in 1865, arguing that reflex activity constituted the exclusive basis for the functioning of the entire nervous system and that all behavior constitutes a mere response (usually in the form of a motor act) to some form of sensory stimulation. Simple acts were believed to be controlled by spinal reflexes, while such complex behaviors as emotions and thoughts were attributed to the functioning of cerebral or psychic reflexes.

Ivan Pavlov built upon the work of Sechenov, demonstrating that reflexive responses (salivation, for example) can be conditioned to such environmental stimuli as the sound of a bell. The environmental stimulus is, in turn, associated with some actual physiological stimulus, such as the sight or smell of food. Pavlov observed, however, that while the sight of food causes salivation, the response ultimately ceases if the animal is not allowed to eat the food it is shown. This discovery gave rise to the concept of extinction, which has broad theoretical ramifications for the study of behavior. The findings of Pavlov have enjoyed wide acceptance, particularly among behavioristic psychologists, who view the mechanism of conditioning as the fundamental element in all learning.

Following the discovery of the structural basis of reflex activity, research in neurophysiology actively centered on the attempt to decipher the mechanisms governing the workings of the nerves themselves. Until the middle of the nineteenth century, neurophysiologists adhered to the classical teachings of Galen, which held that nerves were hollow vessels conveying the animal spirits from the mind to the muscles, thus effecting voluntary movement. It was not until 1775 that Albrecht Haller first discovered the phenomenon of irritability and provided empirical evidence which proved that nerves are not hollow conduits, but constitute instead specialized tissue that responds to chemical and physical stimulation. The discovery of the principle of irritability laid the groundwork for improved understanding of the actual mechanism of nerve conduction, particularly in light of the discoveries made in the area of electrophysiology. Luigi Galvani is credited with discovering the electrical basis of nerve and muscle action through his observation that contacting a muscle with two different metals causes it to contract. Galvani's observations touched off a heated controversy: do nerve and muscle tissue themselves actually possess electrical properties or are they instead passively responding to external stimulation?

It remained to Emil du Bois-Reymond in 1848 to resolve this controversy by demonstrating the resting electrical potential in nerve and muscle, a finding which led to the discovery of the action potential itself. Du Bois-Reymond argued that the resting potential in the nerve results from the migration of electrically charged ions (electromotive particles). These findings did much to dispel the medieval concepts surrounding neurological transmission and marked the transition from dependence upon metaphysical concepts to reliance upon the principles of physics and chemistry to account for the phenomena of nerve conduction.

A key breakthrough in furthering comprehension of the physical basis of nerve transmission was the membrane theory of nerve conduction. In 1866, Julius Bernstein demonstrated the presence of a selectively permeable membrane in the nerve fiber which, when in the resting or polarized state, separates the internal potassium ions from the external sodium ions. (These ions are identical to the electromotive particles hypothesized by du Bois-Reymond.) Bernstein was the first to prove that the nerve impulse is actually a self-propagating wave of negativity resulting from the depolarization of the resting membrane. (Depolarization occurs when membrane permeability changes.)

Bernstein's findings clarified the physical basis of neurological transmission. The work of Keith Lucas, published in 1909, led to the discovery of two important neurological phenomena which have a critical bearing upon behavior and learning. The first was the discovery of the all-or-none principle of neuronal excitation. A given neuron will either fire fully or remain silent because, once stimulated, the amplitude (intensity) of the resultant action potential will always be the same, regardless of the intensity of the stimulus. If a stimulus is not strong enough to depolarize the membrane, no action potential will result. The all-or-none principle states that no matter how strong or weak a given stimulus, the resultant action potentials will be identical. (See Chapter 6 for a discussion of the functional aspects of the action potential in motor learning.) The discovery of the all-or-none principle gave rise to the realization that the nervous system functions in a binary fashion, and ultimately led to the application of cybernetic or control system models to human performance. (The rationale for this approach rests in the fact that computers and the nervous system process information, and both function in a binary fashion.)

Lucas' second major finding was the discovery of the refractory period which immediately follows the excitation of a neuron. The refractory period consists of two phases: the absolute and the relative. During the absolute refractory period, the chemical balance between sodium and potassium is undergoing restoration to the levels present prior to excitation. The membrane is being "recharged" and reset to its initial ready state, known as the resting membrane potential, and no stimulus, regardless of intensity, can elicit an action potential. Following the absolute refractory period is a phase in which the nerve can be made to fire, provided the intensity of the stimulus is greater than that normally required to excite the neuron. This second phase constitutes the relative refractory period. The discovery of the refractory period has implication to learning and performance since it sets limits, the space between action potentials, upon the rate with which a given neuron can process information. Lucas' findings have furthered the understanding of the physical basis of information processing in living organisms and have given rise to a body of theory which directly applies these concepts to the acquisition of motor skills.

Just as advances in neurophysiology furthered the understanding of human learning and behavior, progress in neuroanatomy provided an insight into the workings of the brain itself. Between 1825 and 1842, the French physiologist Pierre Flourens, employing precise surgical techniques, identified the specific functions of the major parts of the brain. It was Flourens who demonstrated conclusively that the cerebral cortex is the seat of consciousness and the crux in the mediation of thought and reason. He discovered that the cerebrum is allied to perception and to the initiation of volitional movement.

Flourens identified the medulla as the vital center of the nervous system, essential to maintaining the life processes of the organism and ordering the sensations entering the brain from the spinal cord. The spinal cord functioned as the conductor of sensory and motor impulses to and from the brain. Among his most significant contributions to understanding the basis of motor control was his discovery of the role the cerebellum plays in the regulation of coordinated movement. Flourens found that if the cerebellum were either damaged or removed, an experimental animal could no longer perform basic motor acts, such as standing, walking, running, or flying. These findings inexorably linked the function of the cerebellum with motor control. Flourens correctly concluded that although the brain is specialized in its functions, all the parts are interconnected and integrated, thus unifying all forms of behavior. (See Chapter 6 for a detailed discussion of the functions and interrelationships of the cerebellum and the cerebral cortex.)

Building upon the work of Flourens, David Ferrier discovered that the cerebellum exerts a regulatory effect upon movement below the level of consciousness. While injury to the cerebellum adversely affects the coordination of muscular actions required in the maintenance of bodily equilibrium, such cerebellar damage exerts no adverse effects upon the elicitation of these movements by the cerebral cortex. Ferrier observed that the effects of cerebellar damage are most pronounced immediately following injury and tend to diminish with time. He attributed this phenomenon to the fact that the subconscious integrative function of the cerebellum is gradually assumed at a conscious level by the cerebral cortex. However, the need to involve the cortex in a process that is normally subconsciously regulated imposes great attentional demands upon the learner and detracts from his capacity to respond consciously to other stimuli. In addition, the conscious (cortical) mediation of these regulatory processes is fatiguing; the organism is consequently more limited in its capacity to sustain an activity. Ferrier's findings apply to motor learning in that early phases of skill acquisition are characterized by the conscious cortical mediation of the activity, the later phases by the automatic regulation exerted by the lower centers. The initial stage of skill acquisition requires greater attention and is therefore more fatiguing than performance upon a well-learned task.

One of the more important discoveries about the basis of motor control was made in 1870 by G. T. Fritsch and Edward Hitzig, who found that motor functions were localized within a specific area of the cerebral cortex and that stimulation of this area resulted in the movement of particular body segments. Using these initial findings, they proceeded to map the motor area and found that stimulation of particular parts of the cortex always resulted in the movement of corresponding body segments. They were able to refine their technique to the point that a given segment of the motor cortex could be identified with a particular group of muscles. (See Figure 6-7)

The findings of Fritsch and Hitzig have given rise to the current controversy concerning the organization of the motor cortex. The basic issue is: are patterns of movement programed within the motor cortex or do specific parts of the cortex innervate individual muscles? In essence, the argument revolves about the question of whether the cortex is organized in terms of the representation of individual muscles or in terms of groups of muscles which work in synergy in the execution of a particular pattern of movement. Since all human movement involves the action of muscles which are antagonistically arranged about joints of the body, coordinated patterns of movement depend upon the alternate relaxation and contraction of these opposing groups of muscles.

J.H. Jackson propounded that it is these movement patterns (e.g., flexion, extension, abduction, and adduction) rather than the individual muscles themselves which are represented in the sensory motor area of the cerebral cortex. However, the fact that an individual muscle is often involved in many movements tends to preclude this type of organization; the same muscle would have to be represented many times over, and such a high degree of redundancy would result in a highly inefficient system. It is currently believed that each muscle is represented only one time in a specific area of the motor cortex and that these individual muscles are simply "called out" as needed during the execution of a given pattern of movement. The system functions much the same as a giant pipe organ—each musical note is represented by either one specific key on the keyboard or pedal of the footboard. The organist creates the chords and the melody through the combination in which the keys are struck and the pedals depressed.

Jackson argued that the reflex constitutes the fundamental functional element of the nervous system, and that complex behavior is dependent upon the patterned integration of individual reflex responses. He further stated that the cerebral cortex is the primary center for such integration and constitutes the locus of the transmission of afferent (sensory) input into complex sensations, perceptions, and thoughts. He believed that such ideational factors as thoughts and perceptions constitute mere abstractions of physical sensations from the environment, and that the integration of such afferent information enables the learner to effect the appropriate response in a given situation. He was strongly committed to the position which held that there is an anatomical substrate to thoughts and feelings, and that many of the sensory impulses which give rise to these feelings (feedback) are the product of movement and physical activity. Once the sensory input has been integrated into higher-order processes, it can be employed in adapting and modifying the learner's motor responses.

While Jackson was a proponent of cortical localization (i.e., he strongly believed that different areas of the cerebral cortex manifest specifically differentiated functions), he also held that these areas do not function in isolation but are, instead, in continual communication. Jackson believed that the major function of the cortex is the integration of the functioning of its specialized areas. Jackson's position is exemplified by individuals learning a complex motor activity, such as a sports skill. The learners modify their response in the light of information generated as a consequence of their actions (feedback). If, for example, they are learning to serve a tennis ball and continually overshoot the service line, they will ultimately abstract the perceived consequences of their actions and, upon processing the information conveyed by the sensory feedback, will modify their response by applying less force on the succeeding attempts.

Although there are still many unanswered questions concerning the role of the nervous system in the learning and performance of motor skills, advances in neuroanatomy and neurophysiology have at least clarified some of the physical bases underlying the regulation and control of human movement and the acquisition of motor skills. Perhaps the individual most closely associated with progress in understanding the neurophysiological basis of the control of human movement was Sir Charles Sherrington. Sherrington (1906) argued that the basic unit of all motor activity is the reflex, since it is by nature a function of innate biological circuitry rather than the product of learning and experience.

In essence, reflexes are prewired within the nervous system and are automatically elicited upon the presentation of the appropriate stimulus. The blinking of the eyes in response to a puff of air and the extension of the knee when the patellar tendon is tapped are both familiar examples of common reflexes in man. All behavior is essentially the result of reflexive activity, which mediates the interaction between an organism and its environment. However, as an organism becomes more biologically complex, the role of individual reflexes diminishes and higher-order integrative activities become more critical. In higher-order animals, reflexive patterns become increasingly conditioned to environmental stimuli, and in humans these complex patterns of association underlie such activities as thinking, reasoning, and learning.

While the behavior of an amoeba, for example, is virtually the exclusive result of reflexive responses to physical stimuli, human behavior, also the result of intrinsic adaptation to extrinsic stimulation, adapts not only to biological stimulation, but to social stimuli as well. The behavior of the newborn human infant is almost completely reflexive in nature (hunger, thirst, satiety). As the child develops, however, responses previously elicited solely through physical stimuli become conditioned to stimuli within the environment. The sight of the parent, for example, soon becomes associated with the pleasurable feelings resulting from the parent's attentions. While the primary ends of such attentive acts as feeding and changing are initially confined to the reduction of the infant's physiological drives, these attentive acts eventually become ends in themselves. In the human, the desire for companionship and social interaction becomes as strong as any of the physiological drives, as evidenced by the fact that an infant will soon cry solely for the attention of the parent, even after all of his physical needs have been satisfied.

A major element in the distinction of human behavior from that of lower-order creatures on the evolutionary scale is that the former is characterized by the capacity to interact with physical as well as social elements in the environment and by the ability to alter the environment volitionally. This transition from dependence upon intrinsic physiological factors to dependence upon extrinsic environmental and societal factors is seen in all forms of human behavior. Proficiency in athletics, for example, is dependent upon the individual's conscious capacity to initiate complex behaviors, which are themselves comprised of co-ordinated patterns of reflexes. Virtually all of human motor behavior is comprised of integrated patterns of reflexes or subroutines which are stereotyped or self-correcting in nature. Running, climbing, swimming, and jumping are all examples of gross motor activities which are volitionally initiated but reflexively regulated.

Although Sherrington's work has provided a basic theoretical framework through which the mechanisms underlying the regulation and control of movement may be objectively examined, his greatest single contribution lies in his recognition of the phenomenon of reciprocal inhibition. This reflexive mechanism causes a given muscle to relax when an opposing muscle is contracting and is central in the initiation and control of any type of coordinated movement. Sherrington's recognition of the phenomenon of inhibition has provided an invaluable tool for analyzing the processes underlying the acquisition of motor skill. The ability of a batter to concentrate on the pitch and at the same time block out the noise of the crowd during a baseball game is an example of selective attention processes which result from the reciprocal inhibition of particular sensory pathways. The player's capacity to swing the bat in a mechanically efficient manner, a skill dependent upon the alternate contraction and relaxation of antagonistic muscle groups, is also a function of reciprocal inhibition. In essence, Sherrington's findings have provided the knowledge of the physical basis of motor control upon which contemporary motor learning theories are founded.

### Psychological Influences

The origins of motor learning have been traced to philosophy and neurophysiology, but it was within the broader discipline of psychology that the area was truly developed. J.B. Watson, rooted in the philosophy of functionalism, formulated the basic principles of the psychological school known as behaviorism. Behaviorism was predicated upon the principle that all learning involves some form of muscular activity and its resultant movement, and that, given the appropriate circumstances, there were no limits to human achievement; anyone could learn anything. It was from behaviorism, with its intense concentration upon movement as the mechanism of learning, that the area of motor learning actually took form.

Although behaviorism's original principle assumed that all learning must involve some form of muscular activity, this extreme position was later modified to emphasize experience rather than movement as a central element. Essentially, behaviorists argue that environmental factors which motivate and reinforce the learner play a far more critical role in the learning process than biological factors. According to the behaviorist position, the proficiency an individual attains in any area of endeavor is a direct result of motivation, instruction, and practice rather than the product of innate capacities. Individuals are far more a product of their surroundings and experience than of their biological make-up. The old cliché, "practice makes perfect," is a prime example of the behaviorist position.

Research in experimental psychology in the late 1800s (which was decidedly behavioristic in orientation) employed motor skills as criterion tasks in learning experiments because the acquisition of these skills readily provided objective evidence of learning. Much of the methodology and equipment employed in motor learning research, therefore, has its origins in experimental psychology. G.T. Fechner was among the first to realize that there is a precise mathematical relationship which exists between the strength of a stimulus and the intensity of a response. He developed methods and specific apparatus (some still currently in use) to facilitate the objective study of perception.

A topic of major interest to experimental psychology and with broad ramifications in the area of motor learning is the study of reaction time. H.L. Helmholtz developed specific methods and apparatus for measuring reaction time and estimating information-processing rates (rate of nerve conduction) in man. In addition, he theorized that the perception of physical sensations, such as vision and proprioception, is influenced by repetition (practice) and prior experience (individual differences).

Of all those who pioneered in the field of experimental psychology, perhaps it is the work of Wilhelm Wundt which has exerted the most profound effects upon the development of motor learning research. Both his techniques and apparatus for recording such factors as perception, reaction time, and muscle strength enabled researchers to assess objectively traits which were formerly confined to subjective, introspective methods of analysis (the verbal report of the subject). Herman Ebbinghaus developed methodology for the objective study of memory and forgetting. He explored the effects of such factors as the length and complexity of the material, the number of repetitions, and duration of nonpractice time upon retention and forgetting. His work has given rise to much current motor learning research into the effects of knowledge of results (KR) upon the acquisition of motor skill. Such issues as the precision of KR and the effects of KR-delay upon motor performance and motor retention constitute contemporary applications of Ebbinghaus' research.

It was within the context of experimental psychology that statistical methods, previously confined to research in the physical and biological sciences, first enjoyed successful application to the study of behavior. From a purely practical viewpoint, these statistical techniques may be divided into two broad classes: relational studies, in which the performance of each of the individuals within a group is compared on different variables (e.g., intelligence and fitness); and comparative studies, in which the performance of different groups of individuals is compared upon a common measure or dependent variable. The application of probability theory, formerly confined to mathematical inquiry, enabled the behavioral researcher to subject the observed experimental findings to rigorous analysis. Although statistical methodology constitutes a powerful research tool, there are inherent limits to its applicability. Experimental findings can never be taken as a direct proof of a hypothesis because they can only show whether or not given results differ beyond the limits of chance. (See Chapter 3 for a detailed discussion of fundamental statistical concepts and their application to motor learning.)

Although research on the acquisition of motor skills was at one time an integral part of experimental psychology, it has since evolved as a theoretical and experimental discipline in its own right. According to Irion (1966), the historical development of motor learning can be divided into three major periods. The first period, ranging from approximately 1890 to 1930, was primarily concerned with defining and exploring the fundamental issues in motor skill acquisition. It was characterized by a highly empirical approach, resulting in a plethora of experimentation but a dearth of theoretical explanation. Research at this time centered primarily upon three issues: massing and distribution of practice, whole versus part instruction, and transfer of learning.

The second period of research ranged from approximately 1930 to 1945 and was characterized by an increased sophistication in theoretical formulations and in experimental design. While experimentation on the effects of practice distribution and studies dealing with transfer of learning continued to dominate, there was an ever-increasing emphasis placed upon developing theoretical explanations for the observed phenomena. As physical educators became actively involved in research on the development of motor abilities and skills in youth and adolescence, the role of individual differences in motor learning was scrutinized more critically. There was a greater reliance upon statistical techniques in skills research during this period. The principles of correlation were applied to studies dealing with the relationships among initial motor abilities, the effects of various conditions of practice, and the acquisition of specific motor skills. A rise in research on the retention of motor skills revealed that the principles which successfully accounted for the learning and retention of verbal information often did not apply to the acquisition of motor skills. The second period witnessed the transition of motor learning research from an area which merely emulated the techniques of verbal learning to an independent discipline with unique problems and specific methodologies.

The third period ranges from the mid-1940s to the present and has thus far given rise to more motor learning research than the first and second periods combined. While such traditional problems as the effects of massing of practice, transfer of learning, and retention and forgetting are still being explored, research interests have expanded to parallel developments in such related areas as learning theory, neurophysiology, information theory, and psychophysiology.

One of the most important new areas of investigation stemming from advances in the aforementioned fields deals with the study of the effects of information feedback and knowledge of results upon motor learning. K.U. Smith argues that information feedback, along with the individual's capacity to process it properly, constitutes possibly the single most critical element in the skill acquisition process. And in addition to the new discoveries concerning the role of information feedback, theoretical advances were achieved in the long-established areas of transfer of learning and distribution of practice. It was realized, for example, that the amount of positive transfer which resulted between two motor tasks was a function of the common factors upon which both tasks rested. The greater the degree of common variance shared by the tasks, the greater the resultant task-to-task transfer of learning.

Perhaps one of the major theoretical advances to occur during this third period was related to the study of distribution of practice, which from its inception was predicated upon the belief that massing of practice exerted a decremental effect upon learning. It was the direct application of C.L. Hull's constructs of reactive and conditioned inhibition to the problems of massing and distribution of practice which led to the conclusion that practice distribution is a variable which affects performance rather than learning. After more than a half-century of research in the area, it was finally realized that the decremental effects of massed practice are transitory and tend to dissipate over time, leaving no permanent effect upon learning.

While research during the third period clarified many of the older, more traditional problems of motor learning, such as the role of transfer and the effects of practice distribution, the greatest contribution is in the broad changes which have been adopted governing the fundamental concepts of learning itself. Advances in the areas of artificial intelligence and cybernetics (control theory) gave rise to a totally new approach to the study of motor learning. Traditional behavioristic theories viewed the learner as passive and focused upon the effects of extrinsic environmental manipulations upon the subject's behavior. Contemporary theories are, in contrast, predicated upon the concept that the individual constitutes a vital and dynamic link in the learning process in that he or she actively operates upon information feedback emanating from the ongoing activity. This altered concept of learning has given rise to intensive research on the role of knowledge of results in motor skill acquisition and has resulted as well in the development of information-processing models of motor learning. These models may represent various stages in the learning process in terms of a series of equations or formulas, some form of schematic diagram or flow chart (as in the case of computer programs), or possibly a series of interrelated geometric diagrams.

However, the mathematical theory currently enjoying the greatest application to motor learning is cybernetic or information theory, which is based on the internal workings of the computer. Since the intrinsic functioning of the nervous system and of the computer is binary in nature (a nerve, like a circuit in a computer, is either "on" or "off"), it is felt that there is a legitimate basis for the application of cybernetic theory to the problems of motor learning.

Proponents of cybernetic theory contend that principles which can account for the functioning of a machine such as a computer, which accurately simulates such relevant aspects of human behavior as recognition and recall, can be employed to explain the behavioral functions of the organism itself. They argue the existence of an array of computer-like information-processing mechanisms within the individual which serve elementary functions in the regulation and control of behavior. These mechanisms, or subroutines, are organized, sequenced, and integrated in a particular fashion when the individual is manifesting a specific behavior. Thus, complex motor activities, such as swimming the crawl stroke, throwing a running pass in football, or dribbling in basketball or soccer, are all comprised of fundamental subroutines which have been ordered and integrated in a particular fashion.

### The Role of Physical Education

Although motor learning is founded in the disciplines of philosophy, neurophysiology, and psychology, it is the physical education profession which has provided a focal point and a major motivating force for current research in this area. Initially, the objectives of physical education centered primarily on the development of organic fitness through highly structured and precisely formulated programs of physical exercise. However, the advent of the progressive movement within education exerted a profound effect upon the fundamental philosophy of physical education and, largely through the influence of J.F. Williams and J.B. Nash, there was an increasing awareness of the social value inherent in physical activity and of physical education as a means through which broader educational objectives can be attained. Above all, there was the realization that physical education is as much a learning process as it is a means for developing organic soundness. Along with this new awareness came the need to understand the mechanisms which underlie the acquisition of skill.

Although the fundamental philosophy of physical education had undergone a major change by the middle of the century, research continued to be dominated by studies dealing with physiological and biomechanical issues. Henry (1956) called attention to the fact that exceedingly little research was being conducted within physical education on the processes underlying the acquisition of motor skills. Rather, much of the research being done fell within the discipline of psychology and was primarily confined to performance upon fine motor tasks. He contended that the methodology and the implications of such studies were relevant to problems concerning the learning and performance of complex gross motor activities, such as sport skills, and that research within the area should be conducted by physical educators. Henry, who is credited with coining the phrase "motor learning," wrote that prevailing ideas of skill acquisition within physical education were based largely upon "armchair speculation" and critically lacked an experimentally derived data base. With his realization that physical education cannot depend solely upon research in related areas if it is to further its own ends, he played a major role in establishing laboratories and designing equipment for the study of the acquisition of the complex motor skills employed in activities such as dance and sports. He realized, however, that such research need not lend itself solely to practical applications in order for it to constitute a valid contribution to progress in the field.

In addition to his contributions to the establishment of motor learning research within physical education, Henry was among the first to realize the highly specific nature of gross motor tasks. He demonstrated that there are no general motor ability or motor coordination factors, and that skill in a given activity is dependent upon the presence of a number of specific abilities. These findings have facilitated the study of transfer of motor learning and clarified the role of motor abilities in the acquisition of complex skills.

Henry stated that the purpose of identifying specific ability constructs should not be confined to facilitating the prediction of a subject's performance upon a particular skill; the main thrust of such research should be directed instead toward clarifying the issue of how specific abilities facilitate the integration of sensory input (feedback) in the coordinated patterning of the execution of complex movements. While the prior knowledge of an ability factor (such as performance upon an aptitude test) can serve as a predictive index for the acquisition of a particular skill, the theoretical value of an ability rests in its capacity to facilitate the processing of particular types of information feedback. Henry's interest in the role of abilities in learning was not confined solely to motoric factors; he was also very much concerned with the role of cognitive abilities in the acquisition of complex motor skills and with the relationships between cognitive and motor development.

Brown (1967), expanding upon the work of Henry, wrote that the bulk of physical education research is concerned with the assessment of physical fitness, strength, and the cardiovascular effects of exercise, and that relatively little has been done in the area of motor learning. While this area has always been at least of peripheral interest to physical education, there is a current need to develop more sophisticated learning models and to further knowledge of the mechanisms which underlie the acquisition and performance of motor skills. Brown, like Henry, was also interested in the relationships between motoric and ideational learning, particularly in terms of the effects of perceptual-motor activities upon cognitive development.

Gentile (1972) further refined the ideas stated by Henry and Brown through the formulation of a theoretical model which purported to account for the processes which underlie the acquisition of complex, goal directed motor skills. Gentile argued that the initial phase of skill acquisition involves "getting the idea" of the movement and depends upon cognitive processes, while the latter phase entails the fixation or automation of the response. Since the acquisition of a complex motor skill is goal directed, the initial phase of learning involves the processing of information feedback concerning the degree of discrepancy between the desired goal of the movement and its actual environmental consequences (knowledge of performance). Based upon the information feedback processed, the learner will modify and adjust the response by varying the intensity and duration (temporal and spatial patterning) of muscular force until the response ultimately fulfills the goal or objective. Some feedback may convey information that is not relevant to the execution of the task, and the learner therefore must selectively attend to the critical cues in the input. This capacity to discriminate between relevant and extraneous factors is particularly important in the performance of team sport activities. In a game situation, the performer often must rapidly process large amounts of information concerning the continually changing environmental conditions (as in the case of the fast break in basketball) and simultaneously screen out irrelevant input (such as crowd noise).

Gentile contends that the execution of complex, goal-directed movement entails the formulation of a motor plan or cognitive directive to which all responses are subordinated. The extent to which the actual performance conforms to the directive of the motor plan is conveyed through information feedback. Based upon this information, the learner is able to make decisions and effect adjustments upon the succeeding responses in order to make them conform more closely to the directives of the motor plan. While the initial phase of learning involves the acquisition of the general concept of the motor pattern, the later stage involves increasing the consistency of the response (number of consecutive correct responses) and refining the response pattern (the form and facility of execution). This latter phase is also characterized by the learner's capacity to adapt and modify the response pattern in the light of changing environmental conditions; the greater the fluctuations in the prevailing conditions, the greater the modifications and adaptations of the motor response pattern.

A recent attempt to provide a theoretical explanation for the processes which underlie the acquisition of complex, goal-directed motor activities was undertaken by Schmidt (1975) in his formulation of the schema theory of motor control. The schema is a flexible motor program which accounts for the learner's capacity to adapt responses to novel situations through the mechanisms of recognition and recall. Although speculative in nature, the schema concept provides a promising approach for increased understanding of the processes underlying the acquisition of complex motor skills.

Adams* (1976), a psychologist who has made extensive contributions to motor learning research, cautions that there is currently insufficient data to support the schema hypothesis and that it cannot at this time provide a viable explanation for the acquisition of complex, goal-directed motor skills. Adams (1971) proposed a "closed-loop" theory of motor learning in which information feedback in the form of knowledge

---

*He distinguished the rewarding aspects of reinforcement in animal learning from its informational properties in human learning.

of results (extrinsic verbal input on such consequences of an act as degree of error) is actively employed by the learner in the continual correction and refinement of the movement. The work of Adams has contributed significantly to the understanding of the dynamic nature of motor learning and has clarified the role of such intrinsic factors as attention, anticipation, recognition, recall, and the systematic processing of information feedback in the acquisition of complex skills by human learners. Adams' contributions serve as the basis for a number of information-processing models of motor learning which enjoy current popularity.

Although writers and researchers in the area of physical education have contributed consistently to the growth of knowledge in motor learning during the last twenty-five years, it is within this past decade that the most prolific and sophisticated contributions have been made. There has been a marked increase in the number of scholarly journals and textbooks dealing with theoretical and applied aspects of motor learning. Although the contributions of physical education have resulted in some significant advances, there are still many unresolved issues. It may well be that the fundamental issues of motor learning are intrinsically so complex that they exceed the capacities of even the most sophisticated experimental methodology currently available.

*Bibliography*

Adams, J. A. "A Closed-Loop Theory of Motor Learning." *Journal of Motor Behavior, 3* (1971), 111–149.

————. "Issues for a Closed-Loop Theory of Motor Learning." In G.E. Stelmach (ed.), *Motor Control Issues and Trends.* New York: Academic Press, 1976.

Boring, E.G. *A History of Experimental Psychology.* New York: Appleton-Century-Crofts, 1957.

Brown, R.C. "Recent Trends in Research in Physical Education." *New York State Journal of Health, Physical Education and Recreation, 19* (1976), 1–4.

Clarke, E. and C.D. O'Malley. *The Human Brain and Spinal Cord.* Berkeley: University of California Press, 1968.

D'Amato, M.R. *Experimental Psychology.* New York: McGraw-Hill, 1970.

Gentile, A.M. "A Working Model of Skill Acquisition with Application to Teaching." *Quest, 17* (1972), 3–23.

Henry, F.M. "Coordination and Motor Learning." *Annual Proceedings of the College Physical Education Association, 59* (1956), 68–75.

Irion, A.L. "A Brief History of Research on the Acquisition of Skill." *In* E.A. Bilodeau (ed.), *Acquisition of Skill.* New York: Academic Press, 1966.

Piaget, J. and P. Fraisse. *Experimental Psychology: I. History and Method.* New York: Basic Books, 1968.

Schmidt, R.A. "A Schema Theory of Discrete Motor Skill Learning." *Psychological Review, 82* (1975), 225–260.

Sherrington, C.S. *The Integrative Action of the Nervous System.* New York: Scribner, 1906.

Turner, M.B. *Philosophy and the Science of Behavior.* New York: Appleton-Century-Crofts, 1967.

Weston, A.W. *The Making of American Physical Education.* New York: Appleton-Century-Crofts, 1962.

Young, R.M. *Mind, Brain and Adaptation in the Nineteenth Century.* Oxford, Eng.: Clarendon Press, 1970.

# CHAPTER 2

# The Theoretical Foundations of Motor Learning

BECAUSE THE ACQUISITION of complex motor skills involves the integration of higher-order ideational processes with reflexively mediated responses, the scientific study of motor learning is contingent upon a prior understanding of the broad theoretical issues central to all forms of learning. A fundamental controversy pertains to the adequate definition of learning; although a plethora of definitions exist, none has achieved universal acceptance. However, it is generally agreed that learning constitutes a behavioral change that can be directly linked to the effects of practice. Changes in behavior that result from the effects of maturation, habituation, or species-specific behavioral programing are excluded from the domain of learning. Habituation entails a simple rise in a sensory threshold, as in the case of adjusting to bright light, loud noise, or noxious odor. A swimmer feels cold upon initial immersion but quickly becomes habituated to the temperature of the water. Species-specific responses pertain to those behaviors that are biologically rooted within an organism, such as the capacity for language in man or song in birds.

Of all the factors that can modify behavior, however, maturation is regarded as the single greatest competitor to learning. The key distinction between these two processes lies in the fact that learning involves behavioral changes which result from practice, whereas maturation involves behavioral changes which ensue over the course of time alone. Although practice will facilitate the acquisition of specific responses, such as motor skills, it exerts little or no effect upon the development of the fundamental organismic traits which underlie the capacity to perform those skills. A classic example of the respective roles of learning and maturation in human behavior can be found in language acquisition. The particular language an individual acquires is the result of learning; the capacity to produce the basic sounds of the language is a function of maturational processes.

However, it is often difficult to separate the effects of learning and maturation, particularly in areas related to child development. If, for example, an individual were confronted with the task of evaluating the effectiveness of a physical education program for the early elementary grades, it would be overwhelmingly difficult and perhaps even impossible to differentiate the respective roles of learning and maturation in the course of the students' progress. Although practice and instruction can facilitate the acquisition of specific motor skills, such as running, throwing, catching, and climbing, the child's capacity for performing these activities ultimately relies on such organismic factors as strength, muscular and cardiovascular endurance, and neuromuscular coordination. The acquisiton of specific skills is directly linked to the effects of practice and therefore constitutes a prime example of learned behavior, while the underlying organismic traits which enable the child to perform a given skill are greatly influenced by developmental and maturational factors. It is reasonable to assume that permanent behavioral changes occurring among students in the elementary grades are the result of complex interactions between learning and maturational processes.

### Behavioristic Versus Cognitive Theory

Theoretical controversy in the area of learning is not confined merely to the problem of definition; it encompasses the very nature and conditions of learning itself. Learning theorists can be classified into two broad theoretical categories: behavioristic and cognitive (Gestalt). Behaviorism is rooted in the objective, empirical traditions established by J.B. Watson, Pavlov, and E.L. Thorndike, and is predicated upon the premise that learning entails either the association of a stimulus and a response or the reinforcement of a response which results through the process of trial and error. Watson (1913), who is credited with formalizing the behaviorist position, argued that since all learning results solely through trial-and-error experiences, it is therefore critically dependent upon muscular activity and bodily movements. Watson's position, however, failed to account adequately for complex, highly organized forms of behavior (such as sport skills) that are directed toward a specific purpose or goal.

Although behaviorism had limited applicability to complex learning situations, Watson remained firm in his opposition to theories which stressed introspective mechanisms or abstract principles as viable explanations of behavior. In fact, he went so far as to deny the existence of thought itself, arguing that thinking is actually subvocal speech, and that feelings and emotions are mere consequences of the contraction of visceral muscles. Since Watson viewed muscular movements as the critical link between stimulus and response, the kinesthetic stimuli (movement-produced feedback) elicited as a result of the learner's activities were regarded as the primary integrative mechanism of behavior. Although Watson's theories have failed to yield a satisfactory explanation for the complex cognitive learning factors involved in the understanding of principles and concepts, they have nonetheless provided a framework for contemporary theories of motor learning.

In contrast to behaviorism, cognitive or Gestalt theory was predicated upon the belief that the critical factor in learning is the individual's capacity to comprehend and organize the elements of the learning task rather than the simple ability to associate a given stimulus with a particular response. Gestalt theorists argue that the acquisition of complex activities is dependent upon the learner's capacity to develop cognitive sets or strategies which enable him to attain his behavioral goal or objective through successful interaction with his environment. As a result of practice and experience, the learner modifies his responses according to their perceived environmental consequences. If a ball is thrown too hard on the first attempt, less force will be applied on the succeeding trial, and eventually the learner is able to adopt the appropriate strategy which will enable him to fulfill the objective of getting the ball through the basket.

Since the study of the acquisition of complex motor skills involves both movement and cognition, neither behavioristic nor cognitive theories alone can satisfactorily account for the processes involved in motor learning. Although many of the issues within this area (e.g., transfer of learning, practice distribution, and knowledge of results) originated as controversies falling solely within the realm of behaviorism, the study of the acquisition of complex motor activities must be viewed realistically in cognitive as well as in behavioristic terms. The general or nonspecific aspects of skill acquisition (principles, objectives, rules, and strategy) clearly lend themselves to cognitive processes, but the acquisition of the specific aspects of motoric activities, which are contingent upon the precise temporal and spatial application of muscular force, is best examined within a behavioristic context.

### Respondent Conditioning Principles

In addition to those theoretical controversies which separate cognitive theorists from behaviorists, there are many issues upon which behaviorists themselves are divided. Advocates of respondent or classical conditioning are rooted in the theoretical work of Pavlov during the early 1900s, which focused on the conditioning of responses elicited by known stimuli, such as an eye blink in response to a puff of air or the withdrawal of a limb from the source of an electrical shock. Proponents of respondent conditioning hold that the central element in all learning is the association between a given stimulus and a given response in close temporal contiguity. Even though classical conditioning experiments have been largely confined to simple reflexive responses, advocates of this position argue nonetheless that the contiguous association between a stimulus and a response constitutes the basis of all forms of learning.

In contrast to the respondent theorists, proponents of operant or instrumental conditioning derive their theoretical premise from Thorndike's law of effect and concern themselves with the study of emitted responses which cannot be linked to given stimuli. Operant theorists argue that the critical element in learning pertains to the consequences or reinforcement (either positive or negative) of the response itself rather than to the association of that response with a given stimulus.

Although respondent or classical conditioning represents one of the first truly objective methods for studying the phenomenon of learning, it was developed within a theoretical context which erroneously viewed conditioning as the basic element of all learning. The classical conditioning paradigm consists of an unconditioned, usually reflexive response, which is initially elicited solely by the presence of an unconditioned, usually physiological stimulus, eventually becoming conditioned to a neutral stimulus which, prior to conditioning, had absolutely no bearing upon the elicitation of the criterion response. An excellent example of respondent conditioning is seen in the case of the conditioned eye blink: a puff of air (the unconditioned stimulus) is blown into the eye, causing the eyelid to blink (the unconditioned response). Immediately preceding the air puff, an audible tone is sounded (the conditioning stimulus) which in no way bears upon the elicitation of the eye blink. After a number of pairings, the tone is sounded but the puff of air does not follow. However, the eye blink still occurs, even in the absence of the unconditioned stimulus. The eye blink is now said to be conditioned to the previously neutral stimulus, the tone.

Although the anatomical locus of conditioning is unknown, Hilgard and Marquis (1961) cite evidence to support the theory that the contiguous association between a stimulus and a response is a central rather than a peripheral process. Their first argument is based upon the fact that conditioning can occur even when the peripheral afferent pathway (such as the auditory or optic nerve) has been severed. Even though an organism may be rendered blind or deaf, it is still possible to condition a response to an auditory or a visual stimulus through the direct stimulation of the intact central (cortical) projection of the particular sensory nerve.

The second argument derives from the fact that conditioning results even when the conditioned response is prevented from occurring overtly. Animals paralyzed with curare were conditioned to elicit a motor response even though they were incapable of performing the response during the course of conditioning. These findings indicate that the critical factor in conditioning is the underlying neurological patterning of a skill rather than the physical characteristics (muscle actions) of the movement itself.

The third and final argument is predicated upon evidence which indicates that motor responses elicited by the external manipulation of the involved limb segments (passive movements) cannot be conditioned. Although a teacher will often guide a student's hand in forming the letters of the alphabet or provide physical support to a student learning a headstand, these skills cannot be learned until the student makes an active effort to initiate the movement himself.

*Contiguity.* Critics of respondent conditioning contend that it is merely an artifact of the laboratory, confined to the conditioning of simple reflexive and visceral responses ("muscle twitch" psychology) with no relevance to complex forms of learning. Proponents of respondent conditioning say that, although their experimentation has been confined primarily to the laboratory, their findings are predicated upon a universal theoretical premise—all learning, both simple and complex, is the result of the contiguous association between a stimulus and a response.

Despite this positive argument, research in the area remained confined largely to the problems originally delineated by Watson, i.e., the environmental consequences of simple muscular contractions and glandular secretions. Critics of behaviorism, particularly those who advocated Gestalt theory, argued that its professed objectivity was predicated upon the study of trivial physiological responses which bore no relationship to complex human behavior.

In the light of these criticisms, Tolman (1932) formulated a theory which attempted to reconcile the rigid objectivity of behaviorism with the broad applicability of Gestalt theory to human behavior. Although Tolman was himself an advocate of respondent conditioning, his theory of purposive behaviorism differentiated between the simple, physiological responses characteristically employed in classical conditioning studies and the complex, goal-directed activities which comprise human behavior. Tolman characterized simple muscular and glandular responses as molecular behavior, and purposive, complex, goal-directed patterns of movement as molar behavior. The concept of molar behavior is predicated upon the supposition that any behavioral act (opening a door, throwing a ball, or executing a handstand) has distinguishing properties in and of itself which are independent of the underlying physiological properties. A physical educator is perfectly capable of correcting a student's tennis serve in the absence of any further knowledge of the neurological and muscular processes underlying the movement.

In addition to his findings distinguishing molar from molecular behavior, Tolman was among the first to state formally how important the interactions between the individual differences of the learner and the nature of the criterion task are. His contributions have provided a theoretical framework for many of the contemporary issues within motor learning. The broader theoretical implications of his contributions will be discussed later in this chapter. At this point, however, attention will be focused upon the positions of other theorists who, like Tolman, advocate the relevance of applying the principles of classical conditioning to the acquisition of complex, goal-directed behavior.

As a leading advocate of this position, Guthrie (1952) argued that the contiguous association between a given stimulus and response was fundamental to the acquisition of complex, highly organized (molar) behavior as well as the conditioning of fundamental physiological responses (molecular behavior). In the case of molar behavior, the complex behavioral pattern (response) was believed to be conditioned to environmental stimuli. When hitting a baseball, for example, such perceived environmental cues as the speed and direction of the ball become the conditioned stimuli for the response of swinging the bat. The molar response (swinging the bat) is itself comprised of an organized sequence of molecular responses which constitute the actions of the individual muscles involved in the skill. Through practice, the molecular responses become conditioned to physiological stimuli in the form of proprioceptive feedback from the preceding muscular response and to external stimuli in the form of the environmental consequences of a particular muscular movement. In the example of hitting a baseball, a given amount of muscular force results in a perceptible movement of the bat in a particular direction. According to Guthrie, adjustment and modification of the molecular response constitute the critical elements underlying the attainment of proficiency upon a molar task. This process is accomplished through the association of the kinesthetic feedback attained from the action of a given muscle with the perceived environmental consequences of such muscular activity.

Although a number of theorists advocate the central role of respondent conditioning principles in all forms of learning, Guthrie's position is unique is that it views skill acquisition as an end in itself rather than a means toward the objective study of the cognitive and associative processes which underlie verbal learning. Perhaps Guthrie's single greatest contribution is his belief that a motor response becomes conditioned to the environmental stimuli present when the response is elicited. The response of taking a lay-up shot in basketball will be conditioned to such environmental cues as the player's distance from the basket and the angle from which he approaches the basket. Through practice, the sight of the basket from a given angle and set distance will become the stimulus for eliciting the response of taking the lay-up shot. Guthrie argues that prevailing conditions during the performance of a given activity eventually beome the stimulus cues for producing that response. Guthrie's position concerning the importance of environmental factors in the learning process has exerted a great influence upon contemporary theorists who view the contiguous association between stimulus and response elements as the central factor in learning.

Bruner (1973a), a leading contemporary proponent of contiguity as a major factor in child development, argues that the initial activities of the human infant are primarily molecular in that they are virtually exclusively reflexive and visceral in nature. As the child develops, however, there is an ever-increasing awareness of environmental factors, and eventually these factors become associated with forms of behavior which were previously associated only with physiological stimuli. For example, an infant soon learns to associate the satiety attained from the consumption of the formula in his bottle with the very sight and feel of the bottle itself. Bruner (1973b) contends that sensory-motor development, particularly in the first year of life, is dependent upon the temporal and spatial patterning of the infant's basic units of coordinated movement or subroutines. These subroutines are themselves comprised of ordered sequences of basic reflexive responses that are "wired in" at birth. According to Bruner, the process underlying the development of complex movement lies in establishing a contiguous association between a given reflexive response and a particular environmental stimulus. These associations are then integrated, adjusted, and refined through the processing of kinesthetic feedback information generated by specialized nerve receptors in the muscles and joints. The result is coordinated complex movement.

For Piaget (1977), the very basis of child development is contingent upon extrinsic environmental stimuli producing responses which initially were elicited solely by intrinsic physiological stimuli. While an infant's earliest associative activities may involve the conditioning of but a single physiological response with an environmental stimulus, the developmental process entails the eventual conditioning of a sequence of responses. Piaget argues that it is the increasing complexity of the conditioned response patterns which eventually provides the framework for cognitive development. Piaget (1973) has proposed a model which purportedly accounts for the factors underlying the development of complexly ordered behavior in early childhood. It is his contention that, under the appropriate circumstances, there is a coalescence among several basic reflexive movements resulting in a single, more complex, coordinated, and volitionally induced movement or act of praxis. It is the combination of these acts of praxis into still more complexly ordered patterns of movement that constitutes the fundamental framework of learning. It is theorized that, during the first two years of life, the child's acts of praxis center primarily on the movements of his own body segments. The later stages of child development are marked by an increasing dependence upon environmental factors and result in a more peripheral and decentralized pattern of interaction and responses.

Probably one of the most familiar practical examples of respondent conditioning is the avoidance response associated with the build-up of static electricity in the body. An individual, having walked across a carpeted surface and touched a metal object such as a brass doorknob, receives a painful electrical shock. After a number of such occurrences, the very sight and feel of the doorknob elicit the rapid withdrawal of the hand, even though no shock may actually occur.

While the preceding illustration is confined to molecular behavior, there are many examples of the respondent conditioning of molar behavior, particularly in the areas of physical education and athletics. A defensive linebacker who is apparently capable of reading a play before it happens has actually become conditioned to associate contiguously subtle changes in the characteristics of an offensive player with the nature of the play itself. For example, he may associate certain eye movements of the quarterback with the direction in which the play will be run, or slight changes in the quarterback's body position or muscle tension with either a pass play or a run. Additional examples of respondent conditioning in physical education and athletic situations may be seen in game signals. In baseball, a coach's seemingly meaningless gestures are associated with specific instructions, such as "take," "swing," or "steal." The catcher "communicates" with the pitcher through a set of gestures which, while meaningless to the opposing team and to the spectators, have been contiguously associated with specific pitches by the members of his own team. The signals called by a quarterback, although perceived as a form of random vocalization by the casual onlooker, are conditioned stimuli for precise responses that have been learned through long hours of practice. The whistle signals used by the leader of a marching band during the halftime exhibition are a further application of the principles of respondent conditioning to molar behavior.

Some proponents of respondent conditioning contend that the development of language itself is the mere result of the contiguous association of certain sound patterns with particular entities, behaviors, and perceived experiences. Respondent theorists argue that all forms of human learning, no matter how complex, are the result of responses which, initially elicited solely by intrinsic physiological stimuli, become conditioned to extrinsic environmental stimuli.

### Operant Conditioning Principles

While respondent conditioning is rooted in the principles of Pavlov, operant or instrumental conditioning is linked to the work of Thorndike. Thorndike (1932) was among the first to advocate that learning is the result of a bond between a particular stimulus and a given response. However, his position differed from that of classical conditioning theorists for it was based upon the belief that these S-R bonds could be strengthened or weakened by the consequences of the response itself. This position constituted the basis for the law of effect, which states that activities which result in pleasurable consequences (satisfiers) will strengthen the S-R bonds; activities whose consequences are perceived as unpleasant (annoyers) will result in their weakening. Upon the realization that reward and punishment do not necessarily exert equal and opposite effects on the strength of learning,* Thorndike modified the law of effect. Although the role of reward and punishment in learning is not as clearly defined as Thorndike had originally believed, the law of effect nonetheless is the contemporary conceptual basis of positive and negative reinforcement.

The law of effect proved highly applicable to contemporary learning theory, and Thorndike proposed two additional laws of learning: the law of readiness and the law of practice. The law of readiness pertains to the learner's capacity to process the information essential to the execution of a task at a given time. If an individual is "ready" for a particular activity, the performance of that activity results in positive or satisfying consequences. A football player who is highly motivated and "set" for the game receives satisfaction from playing in that game. Conversely, an individual who is ready for a particular activity but is denied the opportunity to engage in it will develop feelings of frustration and annoyance. A gifted student denied the opportunity to do creative and stimulating work will often become bored and frustrated in the classroom. The law of readiness applies in the case of an individual placed in a situation that exceeds his or her capacity. For example, a

---

* Reward consistently strengthens a response, punishment exerts little or no effect upon weakening it.

well-meaning parent or grandparent may buy a highly sophisticated toy requiring skills and knowledge beyond the abilities of the child for whom it is intended. Instead of enjoying the gift, the child becomes angry and frustrated when he tries to use it.

Just as the law of effect has given way to the concepts of positive and negative reinforcement, the law of readiness has been superseded by the principles of motivation and maturation. The law of readiness was an attempt to relate an individual's pretask abilities to the acquisition of specific skills. Thorndike's early recognition of the existence of such individual differences prompted intensive investigation into the role of such pretask factors as motivation, maturation, and ability in learning and performance.

Thorndike's third law, the law of exercise, originally stated that proficiency will develop in direct proportion to the amount of practice. He modified this position, however, upon the realization that practice can only benefit learning when a given trial is reinforced with the knowledge of its results, thus providing the learner with information feedback which describes the degree of success or failure in that attempt. For example, a teacher tells a student that the reason he failed to hold a handstand is because he kicked up with too much force. A student left to practice a skill in the absence of such reinforcing information feedback, particularly during the initial stages of learning, will continually repeat the same errors and make no perceptible improvement in performance. The law of exercise is therefore valid only as a corollary to the law of effect since the degree of proficiency ultimately attained is a function of the reinforcing effects of information feedback rather than the sole consequence of the amount of practice.

*Reinforcement.* Operant theorists hold that the critical element in learning is not the contiguous association of the stimulus and the response, but rather the reinforcement of the response itself. Reinforcement is empirically defined as anything that increases the probability of reoccurrence of the response immediately preceding the reinforcement. The basic premise of operant theory states simply that what is reinforced is learned.

There are three classifications of reinforcement: positive, negative, and non-reinforcement. Positive reinforcement is usually perceived by the learner as something rewarding which increases the probability of reoccurrence of the response; negative reinforcement is usually perceived as a form of punishment which increases the probability of making a different response; and non-reinforcement produces no perceivable consequences of the behavior preceding the non-reinforcement. In effect, nothing happens as a result of the response. Negative reinforcement and punishment are technically distinct entities in that the former precedes rather than follows the response. When a negative reinforcer is removed from a situation—dimming a bright light or lessening a noxious sound—the probability of eliciting the desired response is heightened. Since the procedures associated with negative reinforcement require the highly controlled facilities of a laboratory, the technically precise definition of negative reinforcement unfortunately bears little relevance to practical learning situations.

Accepting the operant theorists' position that what is reinforced is learned, one may see that if reinforcement occurs in a random, uncontrolled fashion, the probability of learning an incorrect response is equal to the probability of learning a correct one. This phenomenon is most evident in physical education. For example, a student learning to shoot a basketball with no formal instruction adopts any method, no matter how poor, which is reinforced by the sight of the ball going through the net. A student receiving reinforcement after concluding a series of correctly executed operations with an incorrect response is just as likely to learn the wrong response as he is likely to learn the correct one. A critical element in operant conditioning, then, is timing. If the physical educator wishes to utilize some form of reinforcement in his teaching methodology, it must occur *immediately* following the elicitation of the criterion response.

Up to this point, nothing has been said about the role of non-reinforcement in the acquisition of motor skills. An act which is not reinforced results in no perceivable consequences. An example of non-reinforcement is that of a blindfolded individual who is instructed to throw a ball at a target. The subject is unaware of the distance and location of the target and has no basis for evaluating the success or failure of each attempt. In such a situation, practice is meaningless, as the learner has no basis for adjusting and modifying his response. Behavior that is not reinforced eventually becomes extinct, or otherwise stated, non-reinforced practice results in the cessation of the response. Non-reinforcement is employed in practice situations whose goal is to eliminate certain forms of undesirable behavior: a teacher deliberately attempting to ignore a disruptive student or a parent ignoring a child who is having a temper tantrum. Non-reinforcement is often difficult to achieve except under highly controlled conditions since it entails the complete deprivation of the knowledge of a particular behavioral act's consequences.

Proponents of operant conditioning argue that it is possible to "shape" or control the behavior of an individual through a comprehensive system of reinforcement. A rudimentary example of behavior shaping is seen in the child's game of "hot and cold." The object of the game is for the player who is "it" to find something that has been hidden in the room. As the player gets closer to the object, the other players positively reinforce his actions by repeatedly and rapidly shouting "hot!" If, however, the player begins to move away from the concealed object, the other players negatively reinforce his actions by shouting "cold!" According to operant theorists, it is possible to shape all forms of behavior, desirable and undesirable, through a system of appropriate reinforcements.

A major concern among operant theorists relates to the amount of reinforcement necessary to influence behavior. The consensus is that one should employ the minimal amount that will work. If elaborate rewards are presented, students come to expect these as a matter of course. Any decrease in the magnitude of reinforcement is perceived as a "cutback" from the expected level and is usually accompanied by a decrease in performance. If the educator is uncertain about the amount of reinforcement to be given, his ends would best be served by giving too little rather than too much. Although frequent reinforcement is necessary during the initial shaping of a response, it need be given only periodically after a response is conditioned. Actually, learning that is only periodically reinforced is far more resistant to extinction than learning that is reinforced after every single trial. A classic example is found in the case of gambling, a strong habit in which the reinforcement (winning) clearly does not occur every time. The interest and challenge associated with sporting events are also based upon the concept of random periodic reinforcement, in that no team wins all the time and no individual play succeeds in every instance.

The greatest attribute underlying the wide acceptance of operant conditioning is its simplicity. Its proponents view behavior as a molar entity which cannot be adequately reduced to its physiological parameters. The major argument in favor of operant conditioning is that it works in many instances of complex learning. Its opponents argue that it is too superficial to account for the complex nature of human learning, but its advocates, basing their views upon the fact that operant conditioning principles have been successfully applied to a broad spectrum of human activities, contend that it can be used successfully to modify behavior.

When comparing operant and respondent conditioning, one sees that advocates of the latter position do not deny the presence of reinforcement, but say simply that it is not the central element in learning. Operant theorists argue, in turn, that the stimulus eliciting a particular response is essentially irrelevant, and therefore the central element in learning is not contiguity, but reinforcement. By and large, operant conditioning has received greater acceptance in the areas of learning and behavior modification than has been accorded to respondent conditioning. This is probably due to the fact that operant conditioning appears to have a broader application to molar behavior than does respondent conditioning. The central principle of operant conditioning remains inadequately defined. However, the concept of reinforcement provides at least a quasi-theoretical explanation for many of the observed phenomena of learning.

Although operant and respondent theorists differ upon many fundamental issues, both are rooted in the tenets of behaviorism and share a characteristic disregard for the existence of higher processes involved in abstract reasoning. Tolman (1932), though himself a behaviorist, felt that neither respondent nor operant theory adequately accounted for the more complex human learning activities. He believed that complex learning involves thought, organization, and insight, and cannot be sufficiently explained in terms of either reinforcement or contiguity alone since the higher forms of learning entail more than a mere series of trial-and-error processes.

As stated earlier in the chapter, Tolman was not concerned with the physiological processes that underlie behavior, but instead viewed the study of behavior as an end in itself. This molar approach grew from the belief that complex behavior possesses certain properties that are irreducible to basic biological, chemical, or physical properties. The primary distinguishing characteristic of molar behavior is that it is goal-directed in accordance with objectively determinable ends. Since it is goal-directed, molar behavior is both purposive and cognitive, making use of environmental factors as tools and guidelines in achieving its ends. Molar behavior is, above all, teachable, while molecular behavior (such as a simple reflex) is mechanical and stereotyped in nature. Tolman's theory of purposive behaviorism asserts that an organism is not merely learning movement but is actually learning the meanings and consequences of the movement. Based upon this assumption, Tolman substituted the principle of confirmation for reinforcement in his system, arguing that learning results through repeated confirming experiences rather than as a mere acquisition of habits. If a learner engages in an activity and his expectancies regarding that activity are not confirmed, the probability of his reengaging in the same activity is diminished.

Tolman differed from other behavioristic theorists in that he accounted for species-specific differences among organisms, taking into account the effects of such differences on learning capacity. Lower animals may possess the capacity for conditioned reflex and trial-and-error learning, but complex activities require the capacity for inventiveness and creativity. In addition to recognizing differences in capacity, Tolman accounted for differences in the nature of the learning task itself in terms of its temporal, spatial, and perceptual attributes, as well as its complexity and internal organization. Tolman was also among the first to realize the learning-performance distinction, in which learning sets the upper limit of performance and the degree of learning is thereby mirrored in the level of performance.

While Tolman was concerned primarily with applying the principles of respondent conditioning to higher forms of learning, it remained to Clark Hull to develop an elaborate body of learning theory based upon the principles of operant conditioning. As an operant theorist, Hull (1943) believed that the central element in all learning was reinforcement. He contended that the theoretical basis of all reinforcement lay in the power of any given reinforcer to reduce a drive, whether it was physiological (e.g., hunger or thirst) or psychological (e.g., anxiety).

Hull, like Tolman, was committed to the study of complex behavioral activities within an objective context. In order to achieve this end, he proposed the existence of a body of variables which intervene between the stimulus and the response. In keeping with the behaviorist position, these intervening variables are quantitative in nature and wholly devoid of any subjective or introspective elements, such as feelings, perceptions, or emotions.

Among the many variables in Hull's system, those with the greatest relevance to motor learning pertain to his conception of the learning-performance distinction. Learning is believed to constitute a more or less stable, long-term behavioral state and is regarded to be a function of habit strength ($_SH_R$). Performance, in contrast to learning, is regarded as a function of reaction potential ($_SE_R$), a variable that is subject to large fluctuations due to the effects of changes in environmental and organismic factors. The relationship between learning and performance is critically dependent upon levels of positive and of negative drive states. Motivation or positive drive (D) is an essential intervening variable governing the translation of learning into behavior. The two most critical negative factors involved in the learning-performance distinction are reactive inhibition ($I_R$) and conditioned inhibition ($_SI_R$). The former describes a negative, fatigue-like drive that accumulates with work, the latter, a learned response, such as a "bad habit," which detracts from the overall performance of the activity.

According to Hull (1952), the level of performance at any temporal point can be adequately expressed by the formula: $_SI_R = (_SH_R \times D) - (_SI_R$

+ $I_R$). Stated verbally, this expression implies that an individual's level of performance is a function of degree of learning and motivation, less the level of reactive and conditioned inhibition. Superior performers are characterized by high levels of learning and motivation and by very low levels of reactive and conditioned inhibition. The more motivated the learners, the longer they can practice without accumulating excessive levels of $I_R$. Conversely, students of low motivation and little knowledge are highly prone to accumulating $I_R$. This is best evidenced by the fact that novice performers tend to have a far more limited concentration span than that of highly proficient performers. Varsity athletes can practice far longer and far more intensely than can recreational athletes.

Hull argues that variables which influence learning must exert a lasting effect upon behavior. Such variables as motivation, amount of reinforcement, and distribution of practice are characteristically transitory in their effects upon behavior and are prime examples of variables which affect performance rather than learning. The strength of learning itself is measured in terms of two factors: resistance to extinction and response latency. The better a task is learned, the greater its resistance to being forgotten through lack of use. The greater the degree of mastery achieved in a task, the less time and fewer trials it will take to complete the task. An individual who has thoroughly mastered the skill of bicycle riding or swimming, for example, may go for prolonged periods without practice and yet manage to retain a considerable level of proficiency in the activity. The greater the level of learning attained, the more quickly and efficiently the skill is executed in terms of minimizing the number of erroneous and spurious responses while maximizing the number of correct responses.

Although much of Hull's theory has proven inadequate as an explanation of complex human learning, his clarification of the learning-performance distinction has had a considerable impact upon the study of motor learning. Variables, such as length and distribution of practice, serial order of learning, and amount of reinforcement, which were previously regarded as factors affecting learning, are now believed to affect only performance. With the decline in popularity of Hullian theory, Skinner (1938) became the leading proponent of operant conditioning. Unlike Hull, however, Skinner was basically antitheoretical in his approach, concentrating upon the observation of lawful relationships between different schedules of reinforcement and their respective effects upon learning.

The parameters of reinforcement can be defined along a number of dimensions. For example, reinforcement can be intrinsic or extrinsic, response contingent or noncontingent, continuous or intermittent. It is this variegated nature of reinforcement which makes it suitable to a broad range of specific behavioral applications. Certain motor activities are characterized by high levels of inherent or intrinsic reinforcement, an attribute which can be a valuable adjunct to acquisition, yet counter-productive to the attainment of an advanced degree of proficiency.

The methods employed by the self-taught bowler may be grossly ineffectual; they are nonetheless reinforced every time he succeeds in knocking down even a single pin. If one is concerned with teaching the proper techniques of bowling, reinforcement must be made contingent solely upon such factors as the form of the approach and the release of the ball. Given the high degree of intrinsic reinforcement associated with bowling, this clearly is not a simple task. Powerful extrinsic reinforcement in the form of verbal praise or criticism must be utilized and made contingent upon the quality of the techniques employed. During the initial stages of acquisition, such extrinsic reinforcement must be given following each trial. As the learner develops proficiency, the extrinsic reinforcement need be given only intermittently. Ultimately, the inherent reinforcing properties of the activity become conditioned to the appropriate techniques which were themselves initially shaped and refined through extrinsic reinforcement. The end result requires that the intrinsic reinforcement become contingent upon the elicitation of the appropriate response pattern.

Dickinson (1977) writes that athough sports activities are characterized by high levels of intrinsic reinforcement, there is a considerable degree of interindividual variation in perceiving precisely which aspects of sports participation are reinforcing. Such perceptions vary along a broad spectrum which ranges from the satisfaction derived by a novice performer upon the successful acquisition of new skills to the fame and recognition accorded to the world-class athlete upon securing a major victory in international competition. Dickinson states that the great subjectivity associated with reinforcement in sports is attributable to individual differences in the motives of the participants as well as to the cultural values espoused by a given society. In a cultural milieu which exalts sport, athletic prowess is perceived as a positive social asset; there is no distinction between the good athlete and the good citizen. In societies which place a lesser emphasis upon organized athletic competition, reinforcement is derived largely from the satisfaction associated with self-improvement through the acquisition of new knowledge.

*Schedules of Reinforcement.* Reinforcement can be continuous or intermittent in nature. Whereas continuous reinforcement occurs following every correct response, intermittent reinforcement occurs on a schedule based upon either time or number of correct responses.

Continuous reinforcement is valuable during the initial stages of learning, particularly in the acquisition of complex activities which must be broken down into simpler responses. In this type of learning situation, the partial responses are continually reinforced in an attempt to lead the learner into performing the complete criterion response. In teaching the arm movements involved in swimming the crawl stroke, the instructor may reinforce a response which, while far from perfect, is still a purposive movement bearing some overt resemblance to the criterion response in terms of timing, force, and direction. Through the continuous reinforcement of such partial responses, the learner's behavior is directed and "shaped" until the criterion response is ultimately correctly executed.

Even though continuous reinforcement is a valuable tool during the initial acquisition of a task, few activities in life are continually reinforced. No batter gets a hit every time he is up, nor does a bowler score a strike with every ball. In order to make the principles of operant conditioning more applicable to practical learning situations, Ferster and Skinner (1957) have studied the effects of intermittent reinforcement schedules upon learning. There are four basic schedules of intermittent reinforcement: fixed-interval, variable-interval, fixed-ratio, and variable-ratio. Each of these schedules has particular strengths and weaknesses in terms of its effect upon behavior. Although developed from the response patterns of lower animals and under highly controlled laboratory conditions, these intermittent schedules exert behavioral effects which are relevant to many aspects of human endeavor.

In a fixed-interval schedule, reinforcement is given at set time periods (e.g., every one, three, or five minutes), automatically and wholly independent of the rate of response, i.e., the reinforcement is not contingent upon the response. The major shortcoming of the fixed-interval schedule is that a reinforcement is always followed by a set period of non-reinforcement, with a resultant marked decrease in response rate following each reinforcement. A practical example of the effects of fixed-ratio reinforcement is the supervisor who makes periodic checks on his or her subordinates at the same time every day. The workers will be most productive immediately preceding and during the visit, but will tend to become more lax in their duties in the period between visits.

The variable-interval schedule employs an average rather than a fixed rate of reinforcement. The schedule may provide an average of one reinforcement every five minutes; the time between each individual reinforcement varies randomly from a few seconds to many minutes. (As in the fixed-interval schedule, reinforcement is not contingent upon the response.) The variable-interval scale yields behavior that is characterized by high levels of stability and uniformity and a great resistance to extinction. A practical application of the variable-interval scale is the supervisor who makes random periodic checks on his or her subordinates. Given that the likelihood of the supervisory visit is equally probable at any moment, the workers are far more likely to sustain a uniform level of work output than they would under a regularly timed system.

In a fixed-ratio schedule, reinforcement occurs following a set number of responses rather than a fixed interval of time, so that here, reinforcement is contingent upon the response. Skinner reports that when this schedule is employed systematically (i.e., high levels of non-reinforced responses are approached in a gradual manner), the less frequent the reinforcement, the higher the rate of response. A practical application of this apparently paradoxical phenomenon is used by the demanding coach who exacts very high levels of performance from his players but rarely gives compliments. On the assumption that the players' motivational level is high, the performance level will be maximal when the frequency of reinforcement is minimal.

In the variable-ratio schedule, reinforcement is given after an average, rather than a fixed number of trials, with reinforcement contingent upon the response. Although there may be an average rate of one reinforcement for every ten responses, each reinforcement occurs randomly. It is possible for two consecutive responses to be reinforced, or there may be a large number of non-reinforced responses intervening between reinforced trials. A classical application of the variable-ratio schedule to human learning is found in gambling. An individual playing a slot machine will continue to do so at a rapid, steady pace over prolonged periods of time, sustained by the knowledge that the device must eventually "pay off."

### Cybernetic Principles

Although the principles of operant and respondent conditioning appear applicable to many aspects of human behavior, critics of these theories argue that neither the mere association between a stimulus and a response nor the reinforcement of a response itself is adequate to explain the intricacies of complex behavioral activities. K.U. Smith, an outspoken critic of both respondent and operant conditioning, argues that human learning requires continuous intrinsic regulation and control. According to Smith (1966), the learner becomes a control system between the stimulus and the response. Complex learning activities involve continuous adjustment and modification on the part of the learner based upon information feedback. Since both forms of conditioning involve extrinsic manipulation of the learning situation, they are confined to extremely simple, reflexive modes of behavior which tend to be artifacts of the laboratory, rather than characteristic examples of human behavior.

Smith's views are rooted in the principles of cybernetics, an area concerned with the nature of control processes in biological and mechanical systems. While the traditional S-R paradigms of learning are predicated upon the assumption that behavior consists of a series of discrete, open-loop responses which can be explained in terms of contiguity or reinforcement, cybernetic theories assume that behavior constitutes a dynamic, closed-loop process which is critically dependent upon a continuous flow of information feedback. Wiener (1948) defines feedback as information on the discrepancy between the desired outcome of an activity (e.g., holding a handstand) and the actual outcome (overbalancing). Smith's definition views feedback as a kind of reciprocal interaction between two or more events in which a secondary action is generated which, in turn, redirects the primary activity. Thus, a student shooting an arrow at a target will modify his or her succeeding response according to the consequences of the first attempt.

There are three primary functions of a feedback control system: it directs movements toward a stated goal or target; it compares the actual effects of an action with the desired goal and detects errors; it utilizes the degree of error feedback information in order to redirect the system. A practical example of a feedback system is an individual learning to execute a foul shot in basketball. The initial response is directed toward the goal of getting the ball through the basket. If this initial response were excessively forceful and had caused the ball to rebound off the backboard, the performer would have incorporated this feedback information into the response pattern and would then apply less force on the succeeding attempt. Proponents of cybernetic theories contend that the execution of any skilled movement is dependent upon the continuous monitoring of information feedback.

Smith argues that all movements may be classified as postural, transport, or manipulative, and that these movement components are controlled by different levels of the central nervous system.* In addition to specialized cortical control, each of these broad classes of movement is believed to be dependent upon particular types of feedback information for its precise regulation and control. Smith (1970) contends that

---

* Posture is controlled by centers in the medulla, cerebellum, and midbrain; transport movements are under cerebellar and cortical control; fine manipulative movements are mediated by specialized cortical centers.

postural regulation depends upon feedback information concerning body position in relation to gravitational forces; transport movements upon kinesthetic or proprioceptive feedback; manipulative movements upon extrinsic feedback related to the properties of the object being manipulated (e.g., size, weight, and texture). Complex movement patterns—catching, kicking, throwing, standing, running—are themselves dependent upon the integration of postural, manipulative, and transport movement components.

Cybernetic analysis of behavior focuses upon the integrative action of the nervous system in learning and performance. Smith argues that conventional learning theories have revolved around the temporal relationships between stimulus and response (exemplified by S-R contiguity and the effects of delayed reinforcement), whereas a true understanding of the processes of motor learning requires a knowledge of the spatial relationships governing the constituent elements of the criterion task itself. The author contends that individual movements are integrated into movement patterns through the functioning of a series of interconnecting feedback loops which process information on the spatial relationships among the component postural, transport, and manipulative movements. According to advocates of a cybernetic theory of learning, the central factor underlying skill acquisition is neither such extrinsic factors as the association between a given stimulus and response, nor the reinforcement of a discrete response, but rather the learner's capacity to interact dynamically with the environment through actively processing and integrating information feedback.

The behaviorists' traditional view of learning as an open-ended process in which association or reinforcement ensues is viewed by Smith as a closed-loop paradigm in which the learner is continuously adjusting his responses based upon information feedback. A critical difference which distinguishes cybernetic learning theory from respondent and operant theory is the dynamic nature of cybernetic theory itself. Stimulus information is viewed as input, the subject's response as output, and the subject as the critical link in the control system. It is the learner who must make continuously variable adjustments based upon information feedback or knowledge of the results of the output. Such feedback or knowledge of results then modifies the input, which in turn alters the output. It is essentially this dynamic interaction of input, output, and information feedback that distinguishes Smith's view of learning from those of the operant and respondent theorists. (Chapter 8 discusses in depth the role of information feedback in the acquisition and performance of complex motor skills.)

A student learning the headstand is an example of cybernetic theory in action. The execution of the headstand depends upon the continuous regulation of the body's position in order to counterbalance the effects of gravity. When the body begins to overbalance (the input), muscular force is exerted in the opposite direction (the output). If such force is continually exerted, however, the body will begin to underbalance, and muscular force will have to be applied in the opposite direction. The alternating exertion of muscular force by opposing groups of muscles is characteristic of all skilled movements. The precise regulation and control of these movements comes from feedback information concerning the position and speed of the various body segments involved in the activity. Even the maintenance of posture relies upon a form of closed-loop behavior which offers continuous and varying resistance to the pull of gravity upon the body by the antigravity muscles. These muscular contractions are dependent upon feedback information generated in the muscles, joints, and tendons, and are continually occurring whenever upright posture is maintained.*

Adams (1971) furthered the application of cybernetic principles to skill acquisition by formulating a closed-loop theory of motor learning. He argued that although feedback is a central factor in the learning and performance of motor skills, the learner must develop an internalized reference model or perceptual trace in order to process the information feedback actively and to effect the appropriate adjustments in the ongoing response. The perceptual trace is hypothesized to contain coded information pertinent to the sequential pattern of responses associated with the correct execution of the ongoing task. If the wrong skills are practiced, the wrong model will be internalized. Any discrepancy between the information conveyed by feedback from the ongoing movement and that contained in the perceptual trace is perceived as an error signal. The learner must modify his or her response in order to eliminate the perceived mismatch. The perceptual trace is deemed critical to the regulation of the ongoing response.

Adams (1976) hypothesized a second factor, the memory trace, which initiates a given response sequence. He holds that the memory trace functions as a limited motor program which elicits the correct response under the appropriate circumstances. Thus, though advocating a closed-loop model in the regulation and control of movements, Adams acknowledges, albeit to a limited degree, the role of open-loop processes in their selection and initiation. He cautions, however, that there is insufficient evidence to support the contention that complex, prepro-gramed movement sequences can govern goal-directed motor activities

---

* These responses are physiologically known as the myotatic stretch reflex.

in the total absence of information feedback. (See Chapters 8 and 9 for discussion of the implications of Adams' theory.)

### Task Taxonomy

In reviewing the discussion of learning theory to this point, one can see that all are applicable to all forms of learning, but certain positions provide more satisfactory explanations of the complex processes involved in motor learning than others. The work of Fitts, and thereafter Fleishman, has particular relevance to the acquisition of motor skills. Fitts (1964) has made highly significant theoretical contributions that ramify throughout all aspects of motor learning. He was among the first to realize the importance of task taxonomy, and he identified such task-specific factors as complexity (a factor dependent upon the number of different responses required in the execution of a specific task), coherence (the degree to which a task adheres to a predictable or consistent pattern from its beginning to its end), and continuity (the extent to which a task proceeds in a continuous manner).

In addition to identifying these factors of task taxonomy, Fitts discovered their dynamic interaction with such conditions of practice as massed versus distributed, whole versus part, and practice during early versus later learning. He was also aware of the critical importance of feedback in motor skill acquisition, and he differentiated between intrinsic and extrinsic types. Among the first to realize the dynamic nature of motor learning in terms of the changing factor structure underlying the different stages of motor skill acquisition, he deduced that different levels of skill learning involve different abilities.

A number of Fitts' (1962) findings are also eminently practical in the teaching and analysis of motor skills. His three-stage analysis of motor learning and the nature and conditions of the specific activity peculiar to each stage is of prime importance. The first stage involves cognitive processes embodying such nonspecific factors as the purpose of the skill and the rules and strategies concomitant with its proper execution. It is during this initial stage of skill acquisition that the subject learns what he must do in order to perform the task. Demonstration and explanation are critical at this time. The second stage concerns acquisition. During this phase, the verbal and visual information attained during Stage I are translated into performance: the learner must transform cognitive ideational principles based upon verbal information into controlled movements which entail the processing of proprioceptive information; he must translate words and ideas into information which deals with changes in physical factors such as force, speed, pressure, and direction. It is during the second stage that the transformation of ideation into movement occurs. The third stage is the level of automation: the movements acquired during the second stage are relegated to lower centers of the nervous system and regulated below the levels of consciousness.

Perhaps the greatest practical contribution made by Fitts (1964) to the area of motor learning is his three-level classification of motor activities. Level I activities initially involve a stationary learner and a stationary object, and the temporal pacing of the activity is solely under the learner's control. Examples of such activities are hitting a golf ball, serving a volleyball, bowling, taking a foul shot in basketball, or simply volleying a ball against a wall. Level II activities involve a stationary learner and a moving object and are exemplified by activities such as swinging at a pitched ball or returning a served tennis ball. The temporal pacing of the object is not under the control of the learner. Level III activities are characterized by motion of the learner and the object. Hockey, volleyball, basketball, tennis, soccer, and badminton are prime examples of such activities. Since differences in the nature of the learning task interact with the factors of instruction and practice, methods that are suited to the teaching of Level I skills may not be best suited to the teaching of Level II and Level III skills.

In the case of Level I activities, the learner is able to give full attention to the execution of the criterion skill. In learning a Level I skill, the execution of the criterion task constitutes an end in itself rather than a means to an end. This is not so in the case of Level II and Level III activities. Although an individual may master a forehand stroke in tennis by volleying the ball against a wall (Level I activity), he must then learn to employ the stroke in a game situation (Level III activity) where the pacing is extrinsic. It must be remembered that in the case of Level II and Level III activities, not only must the subject master the skill itself, but must also be able to adapt to the temporal demands of the task dictated by the speed and position of the ball and the opposing players. In teaching Level I activities, there is sufficient latitude to allow for intensive practice on the movement itself, but Level II and III tasks call for an approach which stresses the performance of the criterion skill under conditions similar to those prevailing during the actual game conditions.

Building upon the work of Fitts, particularly in the area of task taxonomy, Fleishman (1964) applied factor analytic methods to the study of motor learning. Although Fitts was among the first to postulate formally the ability-skill distinction in motor learning, it was Fleishman (1967) who strove to identify the basic ability constructs underlying the acquisition of specific motoric activities. Through factor analysis,

Fleishman learned that basic motor ability constructs are divided into two domains, the gross motor and the psychomotor. Gross motor abilities are central to the acquisition of intrinsically-paced skills involving movements of the trunk and limbs, such as calisthenic exercises; psychomotor abilities pertain primarily to skills involving extrinsically-paced movements of the legs, arms, hands, and fingers, as in the case of ball sports. These abilities comprise the relatively general and the permanent behavioral traits accompanying the individual in any learning situation involving the acquisition of specific skills. Skills are differentiated from abilities in that skills involve the application of one or more abilities in the proficient execution of a particular task or group of tasks. For example, the ability of eye-hand coordination is a critical factor in such diverse skills as bowling, shooting baskets, golf, and hitting a baseball. The successful execution of each of these tasks rests, to some degree, in the basic initial ability of the learner prior to its acquisition.

Billing (1980) applied the findings of Fitts and Fleishman to the acquisition of complex, goal-directed motor activities (sport skills) and developed a multi-dimensional analysis of skill learning. He included such factors as the complexity of the environmental stimuli, the nature of the feedback, the complexity of the information-processing and decision-making functions, and the nature of the learning task itself. Billing developed a dichotomous analysis of task complexity based upon Fleishman's precepts of the gross motor and psychomotor domains. He attributes the complexity of gross motor tasks solely to the number and sequential order of the operations that the learner must perform. The complexity of psychomotor tasks, in contrast, is deemed a function of the number of decisions the learner must make and the speed with which they must be effected. In essence, proficiency in activities such as gymnastics, diving, and figure skating is dependent upon an information-processing capacity which is wholly distinct from that involved in the successful performance of team sports.

### Information Theory

Although motor learning is rooted in a theoretical base predominantly behavioristic in its orientation, there is an increasing realization of the complex nature of skill acquisition and a growing dissatisfaction with the simplistic explanations offered by traditional S-R theories. Gentile and Nacson (1976), among the leading advocates of the relevance of Gestalt or cognitive principles to motor learning, argue that despite the profound influence Gestalt theory has exerted upon verbal learning, the role of such cognitive factors as organization and insight has been largely ignored by motor learning researchers. Like Smith, Gentile and Nacson contend that S-R associationist theories are inadequate since they center upon a purely mechanical relationship in which the learner is passive and manipulated wholly by external forces (reinforcement or contiguity). The authors state that motor learning is by nature an active dynamic process in which the learner interacts with the environment through the organized systematic processing of appropriately encoded information. Just as Smith posits motor learning dependence upon the integration of postural, transport, and manipulative movements, Gentile and Nacson argue that the critical factor in skill acquisition is the learner's ability to organize and process task-related information systematically. Gentile and Nacson's position is also compatible with Fitts' three-stage model of motor learning, for Fitts describes the first phase of skill acquisition as heavily dependent upon the cognitive processes of organization and insight.

Although S-R associationist theories continue to enjoy popularity among theorists and researchers alike (operant theory has received particularly wide acceptance), there is a growing belief that such theories are too simplistic to account for the processes which underlie the learning and performance of complex motor skills. In an attempt to reconcile the objectivity of behaviorism with the flexibility of Gestalt theory, motor learning researchers in increasing number are turning toward information-processing models of behavior. These models are predicated upon the principles of cybernetics or control theory.

Such cybernetic concepts as information (in its technical sense), uncertainty, and redundancy enjoy increasing application in the study of human learning, particularly in the area of skill acquisition. Coombs et al. (1970) write that the amount of information conveyed by a message (information feedback) is inversely proportional to the probability of the occurrence of that message (event) from which the feedback is emanating. More simply stated, the less likely it is for an event to take place at a given time, the greater the amount of information generated when and if it should occur. A common example of this phenomenon is the case of individuals executing a well-learned skill, such as jogging, in which the movement proceeds in a relatively automated fashion. If the joggers should unexpectedly step into a rut in the ground or trip over an object in the path, they will be inundated with information about the unexpected event. Suddenly there is a conscious awareness of events that had previously been relegated to lower centers of the nervous system. This concept of information is similar to the neurophysiological processes of arousal in which unexpected or novel events result in the activation of particular centers in the brain.

While the amount of information a message conveys depends solely upon the probability of the occurrence of a given event, the length of a message is determined by the complexity of the event. The complexity or degree of uncertainty associated with a given message can be quantified in terms of binary digits or bits. Since the function of the nervous system is binary in that a given axon fires in all-or-none fashion (it is either "on" or "off" at any given temporal point), the use of binary digits is well suited to human information-processing models. A bit may be defined as the exponential value to which the base 2 must be raised to reach some finite value.

Assume that an individual is confronted with a task that can be correctly executed by selecting one (and only one) of 16 possible available responses. The nature of the task is such that each of these responses falls along an ordinal gradient, in increments of equal magnitude, which ranges between two extreme points. According to information theory, the learner in this example must resolve a message which is 16 words long (each possible response outcome constitutes one word) and consists of 4 bits of uncertainty ($2^4 = 16$). Whenever a learner resolves a bit of information, the length of the message is reduced by half. If the learner is processing information in the most efficient manner, the number of attempts required to "resolve the message" should be equal to the number of bits of uncertainty associated with that message.

Assume that the skill of foul shooting involves a message of 16 words and that on the first attempt the learner throws the ball with excessive force and overshoots the basket. By efficient processing of the resultant information feedback, the learner reduces the uncertainty of the message by half through the elimination of all responses that call for a greater amount of force than that exerted upon the initial attempt. While there were 4 bits of uncertainty preceding the first attempt ($2^4 = 16$), there are now only 3 bits of uncertainty associated with the second, and the length of the message has been reduced by half ($2^3 = 8$). Assume that on the second attempt the learner applies too little force and the ball falls short of the basket. By efficiently processing the available information feedback, another bit of uncertainty is resolved with the elimination of all responses calling for less force than that exerted during the second attempt. This further reduces the length of the remaining message by half ($2^2 = 4$). Following the second attempt, it may be seen that by processing the available information feedback in the most efficient manner, the learner is able to reduce the uncertainty of the message by 75 percent in only two attempts. If the feedback information continues to be processed in an equally efficient manner, the length of the message will be reduced to $2^1 = 2$ following the third trial and to $2^0 = 1$ following the fourth. Assuming that the information feedback has been processed in the most efficent manner and that there is no spurious information to confound the learner's response, the remaining one-word message following the fourth trial ($2^0 = 1$) should represent the correct response. According to information theory, although there were 16 possible responses in this example, the learner was able to acquire the task in only 4 attempts by processing feedback information in a maximally efficient manner.

The principle of redundancy is an important concept of information theory bearing great relevance to human learning. Redundancy involves a departure from maximal efficiency in processing information and is most commonly found when prior experience "transfers" to a current situation, enabling the learner to "save steps." An individual with a prior knowledge of softball will experience far less uncertainty when learning to play baseball than will someone lacking such experience. For the latter, every aspect of the criterion task will be novel and characterized by maximal uncertainty. The greater the consistency of the different parts of an activity, the higher the relative redundancy. The higher the degree of relative redundancy of an activity, the more repetitious and predictable it is.

Driving an automobile under differing road conditions is a practical example of the effects of redundancy upon human performance. Driving on a superhighway constitutes a highly redundant performance situation since the road conditions remain relatively constant for hundreds of miles. Driving on a steep and sharply winding mountain road, in contrast, constitutes a situation low in redundancy, as it is characterized by continuous unpredictable fluctuations in the prevailing conditions. The concept of redundancy, a theoretical explanation for the effects of practice in terms of an information-processing model, is central to all forms of learning. According to an information-theoretic view of learning, practice results in decreased uncertainty associated with the performance of a given task, in other words, uncertainty is maximal during the initial phases of learning but is systematically reduced through practice and experience. However, in certain situations, the level of uncertainty is not affected by the amount of prior experience.

If someone randomly selects a number from 1 to 32 inclusive, and if a second individual is then asked to find which number has been selected, he must always ask 5 questions ($2^5 = 32$), assuming that the first individual has selected the number in a random fashion for each attempt. Regardless of the number of times this activity is repeated, it will always require the learner to ask 5 questions, since prior experience cannot facilitate the performance of the task if the criterion response is randomly selected. With 32 possible outcomes, the first question should reduce the uncertainty by half, and can be stated in either of two ways: is the number greater than 16, or is it 16 or less? No matter which of the two questions is asked, a "yes" or a "no" response (information feedback) conveys an equal amount of information and automatically reduces the uncertainty by half. If the subject has asked if the number is greater than 16 and receives a "no," all possible outcomes from 17 to 32 inclusive are eliminated. Assume that on the succeeding trial the subject asks if the number is 8 or less and receives a "yes"; all outcomes from 9 to 16 are eliminated and again the remaining uncertainty is reduced by half. This procedure is followed until all of the uncertainty is systematically reduced, none remains (a total of 5 questions in this example), and the number is identified. Suppose that the number selected is 6. The message has thus far been reduced from 32 to 8 possible outcomes. Assume that the third question asked is if the number is 4 or less and the answer is "no," once again reducing the uncertainty by half. Then, on the following question, the subject asks if the number is greater than 6 and receives a "no." On the final question, there is one bit remaining, which results in two possible choices ($2^1 = 2$). The subject can ask if the number is 5 or if it is 6. If the number 5 is selected and receives a "no," the same information is received as selecting 6 and receiving a "yes" (namely, that when all of the uncertainty has been reduced, the correct answer is number 6).

If, however, the number is not selected at random but as a result of preference or bias for selecting only certain numbers, or as a result of a tendency to follow some predictable pattern, the learner may be able to identify the number in fewer than 5 questions. The degree to which a task departs from the maximal uncertainty characteristic of random selection factors is a function of the level of redundancy. Old Hollywood murder mystery movies provide a common example of redundancy. Although seeing one for the first time might prove interesting and exciting, the repetitious nature of the plots ("the butler did it") leads ultimately to the conclusion, "If you've seen one, you've seen them all."

Coombs et al. (1970) define redundancy in terms of the formula $R = 1 - \frac{\text{actual uncertainty}}{\text{maximal uncertainty}}$. If a task initially involves 10 bits of uncertainty, but through practice and experience the learner becomes capable of discerning continuities and consistencies within the nature of the task and is able to reduce the uncertainty to 5 bits, the task is said to be 50 percent redundant ($R = 1 - \frac{5}{10} = .50$ or 50 percent). In this situation, the nature of the task is such that an increased familiarity with the organizational processes governing its performance will result in a reduction of half the uncertainty.

The concept of redundancy has many applications to various aspects of human performance. In the area of athletics, for example, the repertoire of a good quarterback or pitcher is characterized by low levels of redundancy since the objective is to maximize the element of surprise and to keep the opposition in a state of maximal uncertainty. Redundancy is one of the reasons a veteran player is less prone than a rookie to make mistakes. A rookie player experiences maximal uncertainty associated with every play; a veteran player, due to prior experience, is able to "read" a play as it is developing. The game situation holds a higher degree of redundancy for the veteran. In every form of athletic competition there is a point at which the performer must commit himself to a definite course of action. The longer this point can be delayed, and the less predictable the ultimate outcome from the preceding movements, the less redundant the sequence and the greater the actual associated uncertainty. A football quarterback deceives his opponent through a series of "fakes." These are often unconvincing to the astute veteran defenseman who recognizes certain telltale elements in the fake. The concept of redundancy is essential to learning, for without it there could be no improvement with practice. In the absence of redundancy, every attempt at performing a given task, no matter how often it has been repeated, would present the learner with the same level of uncertainty as that encountered upon the initial attempt.

Anglin (1977) identified several factors related to redundancy which exert an important role in the child's acquisition of language. These factors, which entail overinclusion, underinclusion, and exclusion, are also applicable to the learning of motor skills. A common example of overinclusion or overgeneralization in the realm of verbal behavior is the child who uses the word "car" to refer to any motorized vehicle, be it a moped or a tractor-trailer truck. Overinclusion can also be found in the acquisition of motor skills. A child will often refer to even the most rudimentary tumbling movement as a somersault. The novice Little Leaguer may regard any contact with the ball, including a foul tip, as a hit, or he may swing at every pitch delivered, regardless of its quality. Underinclusion entails responding to certain objects while ignoring or rejecting others that are in the same logical category. The child may regard spaniels and collies as dogs, but he may not include Great Danes in that same category. In the case of motor learning, the child may regard a round-off and a handspring as gymnastic moves but not include a headstand in the same classification. The novice baseball player may regard only fast balls as "good pitches," failing to swing at all others, regardless of their quality. Exclusion entails the complete omission of a response in a given category. Such omission may be due to inexperience or may result from an insufficient maturational level. For example, a child may never use the terms "carnivore" and "herbivore" when classifying animals. In the case of motor learning, the novice gymnast may never attempt certain moves either because he is not aware of their existence or because he does not possess the requisite physical skills for their proper execution. Although the factors of overinclusion, under-inclusion, and exclusion pertain primarily to redundancy in verbal learning, they are applicable to a number of motor learning situations.

Coombs et al., in addition to discussing the role of uncertainty and redundancy in learning, examine the concept of S-R learning within an information-theoretic context. They argue that a stimulus constitutes a message from the environment to the learner and a response constitutes a message from the learner to his environment. The degree to which a given response is contingent upon a particular stimulus (the degree of S-R constraint) is known as transmission; the greater the probability of a given stimulus resulting in the elicitation of a particular response, the higher the level of transmission. If a given stimulus elicits one and only one response, and conversely, if a given response is evoked by one and only one stimulus, such a result is said to be a pure transmission task. Unfortunately, a given stimulus will usually result in the elicitation of one of several possible responses, and any given response may, in turn, be elicited by a number of possible stimuli. Such a stimulus is known as ambiguous; such a response, equivocal.

In order to ensure a high level of transmission between a stimulus and a response, the degree of equivocation and ambiguity must be minimized. When all stimulus ambiguity is eliminated, the task is referred to as "ambiguity intolerant," and when all equivocation has been eliminated, the task becomes "equivocation intolerant." A task that is both is said to be a pure transmission task. There is, for example, a far higher degree of transmission between a coach's signals (stimuli) and a player's actions (responses) in the major leagues than there is in Little League. Where a young child may experience difficulty and confusion (stimulus ambiguity) in perceiving the coach's signals, the professional athlete responds quickly and precisely (ambiguity intolerance). Common examples of equivocal responses are a false start in a race, an off-side in football, or a boxer's leaving his corner before the sound of the bell. Organized sport activities are equivocation intolerant because of rules which penalize such equivocal responses.

Although the application of information-processing models to the acquisition of motor skills creates a theoretical framework compatible with the structure and function of the nervous system itself, information theory alone cannot cover all the complex processes which underlie motor learning. Each theoretical position provides some insight into optimum teaching methods. Often one theoretical approach may afford the best results in a particular situation, but if the circumstances are altered, a seemingly contradictory theory may afford a more satisfactory result. The learning of motor skills involves many complex interactions between physiological and environmental factors, and no single theory can successfully account for all of the elements involved. However, each theoretical position can contribute to the understanding of specific aspects of this exceedingly complex phenomenon.

*References*

Adams, J.A. "A Closed-Loop Theory of Motor Learning." *Journal of Motor Behavior, 3* (1971), 111–149.
––––––. "Issues for a Closed-Loop Theory of Motor Learning." *In* G.E. Stelmach (ed.), *Motor Control Issues and Trends.* New York: Academic Press, 1976.
Anglin, J. *Word, Object, and Conceptual Development.* New York: W.W. Norton, 1977.
Billing, J. "An Overview of Task Complexity." *Motor Skills: Theory into Practice, 4* (1980), 18–23.
Bruner, J.S. "Organization of Early Skilled Action." *Child Development, 44* (1973a), 1–11.
–––––– and J. Anglin. *Beyond the Information Given: Studies in the Psychology of Knowing.* New York: W.W. Norton, 1973b.
Coombs, C.H., R.M. Dawes, and A. Tversky. *Mathematical Psychology: An Elementary Introduction.* Englewood Cliffs, NJ: Prentice-Hall, 1970.
Dickinson, J. *A Behavioral Analysis of Sport.* Princeton, NJ: Princeton Book Co., 1977.
Ferster, C.S. and B.F. Skinner. *Schedules of Reinforcement.* New York: Appleton-Century-Crofts, 1957.
Fitts, P.M. "Factors in Complex Skill Training." *In* R. Glaser (ed.), *Training Research and Education.* Pittsburgh: University of Pittsburgh Press, 1962.
––––––. "Perceptual-Motor Skill Learning." *In* A.W. Melton (ed.), *Categories of Human Learning.* New York: Academic Press, 1964.
Fleishman, E.A. "The Description and Prediction of Perceptual-Motor Skill Learning." *In* R. Glaser (ed.), *Training Research and Education.* Pittsburgh: University of Pittsburgh Press, 1962.
––––––. *The Structure and Measurement of Physical Fitness.* Englewood Cliffs, NJ: Prentice-Hall, 1964.
––––––. "Individual Differences and Motor Learning." *In* R.M. Gagné (ed.), *Learning and Individual Differences.* Columbus, Ohio: Merrill, 1967.

Gentile, A.M. and J. Nacson. "Organizational Processes in Motor Control." *In* J. Keogh and R.S. Hutton (eds.), *Exercise and Sport Sciences Reviews.* Santa Barbara, Cal.: Journal Publishing Affiliates, 1976.

Guthrie, E.R. *The Psychology of Learning.* New York: Harper and Row, 1952.

Hilgard, E.R. and D.G. Marquis. *Conditioning and Learning.* 2nd ed. New York: Appleton-Century-Crofts, 1961.

Hull, C.L. *Principles of Behavior.* New York: Appleton-Century-Crofts, 1943.

––––––. *A Behavior System: An Introduction to Behavior Theory Concerning the Individual Organism.* New Haven, Conn.: Yale University Press, 1952.

Piaget, J. *The Child and Reality.* New York: Grossman, 1973.

––––––. "The First Year of Life of the Child." *In* H.E. Gruber and J.J. Vonèche (eds.), *The Essential Piaget.* New York: Basic Books, 1977.

Skinner, B.F. *The Behavior of Organisms: An Experimental Analysis.* New York: Appleton-Century-Crofts, 1938.

Smith, K.U. and G. "Feedback Mechanisms of Athletic Skill." *In* L.E. Smith (ed.), *Psychology of Motor Learning.* Chicago: The Athletic Institute, 1970.

–––––– and M.F. *Cybernetic Principles of Learning and Educational Design.* New York: Holt, Rinehart and Winston, 1966.

Thorndike, E.L. *The Fundamentals of Learning.* New York: Teachers College Press, 1932.

Tolman, E.C. *Purposive Behavior in Animals and Men.* New York: Appleton-Century-Crofts, 1932.

Watson, J.B. "Psychology As the Behaviorist Views It." *Psychological Review, 20* (1913), 158–177.

Wiener, N. *Cybernetics.* New York: Wiley, 1948.

# CHAPTER 3

# Fundamental Statistical Concepts of Motor Learning Research

AN UNDERSTANDING of the processes which underlie motor learning depends upon assessing the applicability of given theoretical positions to specific aspects of skill acquisition. The fundamental paradigm employed to achieve this end entails the manipulation of independent variables (e.g., practice distribution, serial order of instruction, knowledge of results) for the purpose of observing the resultant effects upon one or more dependent variables (e.g., rate of acquisition, number of errors, length of retention). This procedure may be informal, as in the case of a classroom teacher trying out a new method and subjectively evaluating the results, or a highly structured experimental design whose findings are subjected to rigorous statistical analysis. Either of these techniques may be effective provided the methodology employed is relevant to the nature of the problem under study.

There exists, however, an unfortunate tendency to equate any quantitative approach to the solution of a problem with the scientific method and the precision and objectivity characteristically associated with it. While virtually any observable aspect of human performance may be quantified, the indiscriminate use of quantitative techniques will confound rather than clarify an issue. If quantitative methodology is to be applied to the study of skill acquisition in a meaningful manner, the values (numerical quantities) employed must truly convey some property of the trait under investigation, for example, its size, weight, or some measure of value per unit time (cycles per second or miles per hour). When nominal values (arbitrary numbers which do not truly reflect any measurable aspect of the entity under study) are loosely used to make the observation of behavioral phenomena more objective, the net result is a body of findings that is unreliable and invalid.

## Measurement Scales

There are four types of measurement scales which can be employed in the study of skill acquisition: nominal, ordinal, interval, and ratio. Each of these scales has distinct limitations and any one scale may be particularly well suited to the study of a specific problem within the area of motor learning. The use of nominal values in motor learning is primarily confined to labeling and identification. Common examples of the application of nominal scales to the study of motor skill acquisition are numbers given to experimental subjects or those assigned to the players on a team. There is absolutely no relationship between the magnitude of a player's number and the ability of the player; the number does not connote any property or characteristic (size, weight, or speed) of the player, but serves only as an arbitrarily assigned means of identification. Clearly, nominal values cannot be subjected to any meaningful form of statistical analysis.

Motor learning often deals with variables which fall into some form of ranked order, and such data naturally lends itself to treatment on an ordinal scale. The ordinal scale possesses the property of transitivity in that it proceeds in either an increasing or decreasing order. Common examples of ordinal data are found in such diverse situations as team standings in a league, order of finish in a race, or a size place line-up of students. Although an ordinal scale can convey the idea of elements preceding or following other elements (first, second, or third), it cannot convey the degree to which these elements differ. In the case of the size place line-up, for example, the ordinal scale simply conveys the idea that any individual in the line is equal in height or taller than the person in front of him and equal in height or shorter than the person behind. There is, however, no way of knowing the rate of height difference between individuals. The rate of change between each element in an ordinal scale cannot be presumed to be constant. If one were considering the order of finish in the Boston Marathon, for example, there would be tremendous variation in the proximity of the second place finisher to the first, the third to the second, the fourth to the third, and so on throughout the entire field of finishers. An ordinal scale can reveal only the direction of change, but nothing about its rate.

An ordinal scale in and of itself can be a valid research tool, and a number of widely used statistical techniques employ ordinally ranked data. For example, the Spearman rho, or rank correlation coefficient, is a statistical technique used to correlate two sets of ordinally ranked data, such as judges' ratings. Unfortunately, there is often a temptation to "further the accuracy" of ordinal data through the assignment of arbitrarily distributed "precise score values." In effect, such scores are merely nominal values and decrease the validity of the findings far more than they strengthen them. The only way in which ordinal measures can truly be strengthened is when the rate of change between each value is known.

If the actual unit or interval of change is measured, an ordinal scale is converted to a more powerful measurement technique, the interval scale. An interval scale, based on units of measurement such as inches or centimeters, can reveal the precise degree of difference in height between individuals, or, applied to the order of finish in a race, the precise degree of difference between first and second, second and third, and so on, based on a measure of time.

An extension of the interval scale is the ratio scale. Although the ratio scale is one of the most powerful measurement techniques known, its application to behavioral measurements is extremely limited. In effect, a ratio scale is an interval scale which has an absolute zero point and thus may be used to make comparative statements. If one student weighs 50 pounds and another weighs 100, it can be rightly stated that the heavier student weighs twice as much as the lighter one, starting from the absolute zero point present on the scale employed to measure body weight. When comparing two scores on a physical fitness test, however, a student scoring 80 points could not be said to be twice as fit as a student who scores only 40 points because there is no absolute zero point at which the trait of physical fitness is completely absent. Whereas ratio scales are applicable to measurements of a physical nature, the interval scale represents the most powerful technique for use in the interpretation of behavioral data.

*Variables.* In the course of discussing the various measurement scales which can facilitate the objective analysis of behavioral issues and basic factors of human performance, frequent reference was made to the term "variable." A variable is a sequence of two or more mutually exclusive categories. Data falling in one category is automatically precluded from simultaneously falling in any other category. An individual running 100 yards in 10 seconds, for example, cannot at the same time run the same distance in 9 seconds or in 11 seconds. In a mutually exclusive situation, any one outcome precludes all other outcomes at the same moment in time.

Variables with only two possible outcomes are designated as dichotomous and are exemplified by situations such as pass-fail grading, true-false tests, acceptance or rejection of a statistical hypothesis, winning or losing, and coin tossing. Since dichotomous variables greatly facilitate the process of classification, even variables with an infinite number of outcomes (e.g., time required to run a quarter mile) may be dichotomized by assigning a particular value as a cutoff point separating acceptable or passing performance from that which is failing or unacceptable.

The objective assessment of complex behavior involves the use of both discrete and continuous variables. The categories comprising a discrete variable are separate from each other and may be counted exactly, as in the number of points scored on a test, number of people in a class, or number of seats in an auditorium. Continuous variables cannot be measured exactly but can only be approximated. Measures such as time and distance are characteristic examples of continuous variables because there is no set place where one unit ends and the succeeding one begins. There is no clear cutoff point between one minute and two minutes: the measurement may be carried to the nearest second, millisecond, microsecond, or nanosecond, but it is nevertheless an approximation.

The categories of a discrete variable are complete units in and of themselves. For example, if one student in a basketball game scores 9 baskets and another scores 10, it would be impossible for a third student to score a number of baskets between 9 and 10. In the case of the continuous variable, however, an infinite number of outcomes is possible. If one student runs a distance of 100 yards in 10 seconds, while a second student takes 11 seconds to run the same distance, it is theoretically possible for any number of students to run this distance in the span of time between 10 and 11 seconds.

Discrete variables are particularly applicable to situations in which the concern is frequency data, data which relates to the number of entities falling within a particular category. The number of registered voters between ages 18 and 21, the number of students in a school's senior class, or the number of people attaining a particular score on an exam are examples of frequency data. Discrete variables are integrally related to frequency data; continuous variables constitute the basis of metric data, which is derived from some actual property, such as height, weight, time, or distance, of the entity under study.

### Central Tendency and Variability

The objective investigation of the acquisition of motor skills has characteristically been confined to two fundamental statistical approaches equally applicable to frequency and to metric data. These are the relational study and the comparative study. Relational studies examine the performance of a group of individuals on two different measures; comparative studies, the performance of two different groups of individuals on a common variable. Although such statistical methods are powerful tools of research, commitment to them invariably results in subordination of the individuality of each subject to the concept of measures of central tendency or average which purportedly reflects the performance of the entire group rather than that of each individual within the group.

There are several values used to reflect central tendency; one such measure is the mode. The mode is a frequency measure which, in its crudest form, is designated simply by the most frequently occurring score. The crude mode is easily computed and is based on the assumption that the most frequently occurring score best represents all the scores in the group. There is a fairly simple statistical formula, $Mo = 3Mdn - 2M$ ($Mo$ = Mode, $Mdn$ = Median, $M$ = Mean) which can be used to attain a somewhat more accurate estimate of the mode.

A second value often employed as a measure of central tendency is the median. The median is also based on frequency and is, in fact, a scorepoint in the distribution occupying the middle frequency and dividing the upper half of the distribution from the lower half. Succinctly, the median is the point at which the distribution divides into two equal parts.

While the mode and the median are both based solely upon frequency values, the mean is the more powerful measure of central tendency: it is derived from the average of the actual metric value of each score in the distribution. For this reason, the mean is influenced to a far greater degree by extreme values than are the other measures of central tendency. Unlike the mode and the median, it is always the arithmetic balance point of the distribution in that the deviations above it completely balance out the deviations below.

All measures of central tendency only indicate the average performance level within a group. The manner in which performance varies around the average becomes an area of critical interest since the greater the variability, the greater the diversity of ability within the group. A homogeneous group is characterized by little variability. The simplest and least powerful measure of variability is the range, which is based upon the difference between the highest and lowest scores within the group. (The greater the difference, the greater the range.)The range is customarily employed in conjunction with the mode, as neither measure is particularly powerful.

Somewhat more powerful than range alone is the interquartile range. Since this measure is based upon the difference between the two respective scorepoints in the distribution which cut off the upper quarter of the group, or third quartile ($Q_3$), and the lower quarter, or first quartile ($Q_1$), it is a more accurate estimate of variability. The interquartile range is, in effect, based upon the difference between the scorepoints cutting off the middle 50 percent of the group and is therefore more representative than is the range. The semi-interquartile range is a measure of variability derived simply by taking half of the interquartile range. The interquartile range and the semi-interquartile range are both used in conjunction with the median, as they are derived from scorepoints cutting off set proportions of the group. (The median is always equal to the second quartile, $Q_2$.) (See Figure 3-1)

## Figure 3-1

### INTERQUARTILE RANGE

| | | |
|---|---|---|
| Upper scorepoint limit | $Q_3$ | 75% |
| of interquartile range | | |
| | | |
| Median | $Q_2$ | 50% |
| | | |
| | | |
| Lower scorepoint limit | $Q_1$ | 25% |
| of interquartile range | | |

$$\text{Interquartile range} = Q_3 - Q_1$$

$$\text{Semi-interquartile range} = \frac{Q_3 - Q_1}{2}$$

$$\text{Median} = Q_2$$

The most powerful measure of variability is the standard deviation, a metric value based on the deviation of every score in the distribution from the mean of that distribution. The derivation of the standard deviation requires considerable computation since it is the square root of the average of all the squared deviations from the mean in a given group. Since the standard deviation and the mean are metric values, they are used in conjunction and are the only values which can be employed when the aim of the study is to draw inference to a broader population rather than to confine the findings to a mere description of the group under study.

### Statistical Inference and Decision

If it is the researcher's aim to apply his data to a broader population, the sample from which the data is obtained must be truly representative of the targeted population. In order to obtain a representative sample, special techniques must be employed to ensure that all segments of the population are given an equal opportunity for selection. Such random sampling techniques are most similar to a lottery in which each subject is assigned an identifying number and the numbers are then selected at random. If the researcher is performing a complex experiment with many experimental treatments, the assignment of subjects to each treatment group must also be done on a random basis. Unfortunately, randomization is frequently confused with arbitrary selection and assignment of subjects. Arbitrary selection and assignment introduce selective errors that bear adversely upon the methods of statistical evaluation. By assigning subjects to groups on the basis of a fixed, predetermined, consecutive order, the principle of random selection is violated since each subject does not have an equal opportunity to be assigned to any given group.

A phenomenon related to randomization is the concept of normality of distribution. Behavioral traits are randomly distributed throughout a population in that the majority of individuals will possess a level of the trait closer to the average value of the population than to any other value. As one proceeds from the average toward either extreme, increasingly fewer individuals manifesting the trait will be found. The classic model of a normal distribution is found in the Gaussian distribution, more commonly referred to as the Bell Curve. (See Figure 3-2) When data is normally distributed and the mean and the standard deviation are known, it is possible to make comparisons between various types of data through the use of standard scores. A standard or z score relates all forms of observed data to portions of the area under the normal curve. This procedure allows for the comparison of many different behavioral traits upon a common standard of reference. Percentile ranking is one of the most common applications of standard score measurements to behavioral research. Since it is possible to assess an individual's standing within the overall population in such diverse areas as motor, verbal, and quantitative activities, the use of these techniques enables the researcher to evaluate an individual in terms of a broad spectrum of behavioral traits.

**Figure 3-2**
**AREAS UNDER THE NORMAL DISTRIBUTION CURVE**

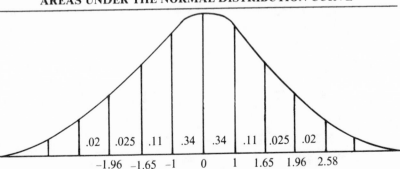

The normal curve also provides the basis for statistical decision in experimental studies. Statistical decision rests heavily upon a concept similar to the American juridical tenet that an individual is presumed innocent until proven guilty beyond a reasonable doubt. Every experimental design is an empirical test of a hypothesis of chance or null hypothesis. The null hypothesis is analogous to the presumption of innocence in that it is regarded as true until sufficient evidence exists to disprove it. A null hypothesis states that all observed differences among the findings, regardless of magnitude, are not significantly different from zero, and are due solely to the effects of chance. The minimum level for rejecting a null hypothesis, on the grounds that the findings significantly exceed the limits of chance, is the 5 percent level of confidence.

If a null hypothesis is rejected at the 5 percent (.05) level, there are still 5 chances in every 100 that, even though it has been rejected, it is still true. A more conservative approach utilizes the one percent (.01) level of significance. If a null hypothesis is rejected at this level, there is only one chance in 100 that it is actually true. Inevitably, there is a question of which level of significance to select, the .05 or the .01. Unfortunately, there is no definite answer, only the choice between belief in something true that is actually false, or something false that is in effect true. In essence, statistical decision always involves the alternative possibilities of either believing a lie or rejecting the truth.

If the findings of a study are actually due to chance, but based upon the evidence the null hypothesis has been rejected erroneously, a type one error is said to have occurred. Referring back to our forensic analogy, this equals a jury conviction of an individual who is actually innocent. However, if the findings of a study are due to some valid consideration or factor other than chance, but insufficient evidence exists for rejecting the null hypothesis and it is accepted although false, a type two error has occurred. These circumstances are analogous to a jury finding an individual innocent who is actually guilty.

The following table will help to clarify the relationships between levels of significance and types of errors.

|  | Type 1 Error | Type 2 Error |
|---|---|---|
| .05 level of significance | 5% | 95% |
| .01 level of significance | 1% | 99% |

It is readily seen that a complementary relationship exists between the probabilities associated with making type one and type two errors at a given level of significance. The most critical factor, however, is that as the odds of making a type one error decrease from 5 in 100 to 1 in 100, the odds of making a type two error increase from 95 in 100 to 99 in 100. In essence, as the odds of making a type one error decrease, the odds of making a type two error increase.

A look at how the findings of comparative studies are analyzed for statistical significance may be useful here. The basic design of a comparative or experimental study involves the comparison of the effects of different conditions of some environmental manipulation (independent variable)—nature and conditions of practice, method of instruction, or schedule and type of reinforcement—upon some criterion performance measure (dependent variable)—time, score, or some measure of distance or weight. An example of the application of experimental methodology to motor learning research can be found in how the effects of practice distribution on the acquisition of a selected criterion skill are studied.

The temporal variations in the conditions of practice (the massing versus the distribution) constitute the independent variable; the dependent variable can be operationally defined in terms of the amount of time or the number of trials required for the initial acquisition of the task. Since the mean value is assumed to represent best the performance of the entire group upon the dependent variable, comparisons are made based upon differences between the means of the experimental groups receiving different conditions of the independent variable. In the preceding example, either the mean time or mean number of trials to the acquisition of the criterion task for those practicing under massed conditions would be compared to that of subjects practicing the same skills under distributed conditions. The actual difference between the means is known as the observed difference.

Basically, there are two conditions that can affect the magnitude of the mean and the resultant observed differences. The first condition is predicated upon the premise that the mean of one group is higher than the mean of another because more individuals performed at a higher level in the group. A second factor is the presence of extreme scores. Assume that a bowling team has scored an average of 100 points during its first year of league play and an average of 125 points during its second year of competition. One explanation for the increased mean performance might lie in the fact that everyone on the team improved as a result of experience. However, a second explanation may well lie in the addition of one highly skilled bowler whose exceptional performance raises the entire team average. As a rule, differences between group means tend to be significant when such differences are based upon a higher overall level of performance in one group than in another.

Conversely, when differences between group means are due to the effects of extreme scores in one group, they tend not to be statistically significant.

The actual determination of statistical significance is predicated upon the ratio of the observed differences between the means of the experimental groups to the variability within the groups. The numerator expresses the actual degree of difference between the group means upon the performance of the dependent variable; the denominator, the range or variability of performance within each group. As with any ratio, the absolute value of the expression increases if the denominator increases and the numerator is held constant. Therefore, upon perfunctory analysis, it would appear that the greater the observed mean differences, the greater the theoretical likelihood of these differences being statistically significant. However, mean differences resulting from the effect of extreme scores are also accompanied by compensatory increases in the variability factors which make up the denominator of the expression. This increase in variability counterbalances the degree of observed difference, i.e., an increase in the numerator of the expression is accompanied by a proportional increase in the denominator.

At this point, it is reasonable to question the actual magnitude of a ratio necessary for the rejection of a null hypothesis at a stated level of confidence. The ratio is not fixed, but varies with such factors as the size of the sample, the number of experimental groups, and the directionality of the hypothesis. In the case of experimental studies employing very large samples of 500 or more, divided into only two groups, and utilizing a non-directional hypothesis, a ratio of slightly less than 2 to 1 is required between the observed differences and the expected differences in order to reject a null hypothesis at the 5 percent level of confidence, slightly more than 2.5 to 1 for findings to be significant at the 1 percent level of confidence. (A non-directional hypothesis states only that the group means will differ beyond the limits of chance, not which group will be superior.) Although there exist far more complex experimental designs for comparing several groups' performance, often upon a number of dependent variables, the tenability of the null hypothesis still resides in the magnitude of the ratio between the differences among the experimental groups and the differences within them.

It is essential that appropriate caution be employed when interpreting the findings of any experimental investigation. It must be remembered that findings which are statistically significant do not necessarily offer direct proof of the validity of the experimental hypothesis but only imply that the observed differences exceed the limits of chance. For this reason, the findings of any given study (regardless of their level of significance) can be taken only as evidence of a particular trend or phenomenon which must be pursued and clarified through further research. The value of the contribution of experimental methodology to motor learning research, therefore, does not rest in the findings of any single study, but is dependent instead upon the results of many experiments, all of which tend to yield consistent findings on a given issue. When a number of researchers are able to replicate an experiment and obtain consistent findings, the implication is that such empirical evidence offers indirect support for a given hypothesis.

### Correlation

Although the preceding discussion has been confined to experimental investigations, studies on the magnitude of the relationship between selected variables are also highly valuable tools of research. Experimental studies are a comparison of the performance of two or more groups of individuals on a common dependent variable. Correlational studies compare the performance of the same group of individuals on two separate measures of performance. The strength of this relationship is determined by the absolute value of the correlation coefficient, which falls between zero and one. Correlation is predicated upon consistency of performance between two variables. When subjects hold the same positions in relation to the mean of the second variable as they do in relation to the mean of the first variable, the correlation is high. (See Figure 3-3) If, however, there is little or no relationship between the subjects' performance on the two measures, the resultant correlation coefficient will be low. (See Figure 3-4)

**Figure 3-3**

**POSITIVE CORRELATION**

| Var. X | Var. Y |
|--------|--------|
| 100 | 600 |
| 200 | 700 |
| 300 | 800 |
| 400 | 900 |
| 500 | 1,000 |

**Figure 3-4**

### NEGATIVE CORRELATION

| Var. X | Var. Y |
|--------|--------|
| 500 | 600 |
| 400 | 700 |
| 300 | 800 |
| 200 | 900 |
| 100 | 1,000 |

**Figure 3-5**

### NO CORRELATION

| Var. X | Var. Y |
|--------|--------|
| 100 | 800 |
| 200 | 600 |
| 300 | 1,000 |
| 400 | 900 |
| 500 | 700 |

A negative correlation results when the subjects achieving the highest scores on the first variable attain the lowest scores on the second variable, and vice versa. (See Figure 3-5) Negative correlations are usually observed in situations where good performance on one measure is indicated by a high score, but superior performance on the second measure is indicated by a low score. If one were to correlate performance upon a physical fitness test with performance on the 100-yard dash, for example, the observed correlation coefficient would most likely be negative because individuals who are most fit should also be fastest, those who are least fit should be slowest. Since speed is the reciprocal of time (high speed means low time), performance measures based upon incremental scores, when correlated with measures of speed, will result in negative correlation.

The magnitude of a given correlation coefficient is indicative only of the degree to which two variables are linearly related (either directly or inversely). It is therefore critical to interpret correlational data with caution, particularly in regard to the inference of causal relationships. If two variables are strongly related (e.g., physical fitness and proficiency in sports activity) it does not necessarily imply that a cause and effect relationship exists between them, but rather that both variables are dependent upon common factors such as strength, flexibility, and muscular endurance, as in the example cited.

The strength of a correlation coefficient is directly proportional to its absolute value since the square of any observed correlation coefficient, when multiplied by 100, yields a fairly accurate estimate of the degree to which the two variables under study overlap. If a researcher observed a correlation of -.90 between two variables, it would mean, first, that the variables were inversely related and, second, and of greater import, that there is an 81 percent overlap between the variances of the two measures. In effect, 81 percent of the factors determining performance upon the first variable are the same determining performance upon the second variable. The higher the absolute value of the correlation coefficient, the greater the amount of common variance between the two variables and the more they tend to reflect the same factors. The higher the correlation between two variables, the greater the likelihood that those variables will actually measure the same thing. (See Figure 3-6) It is precisely this property that has resulted in the broad applicability of

**Figure 3-6**

**TABLE OF REPRESENTATIVE CORRELATION COEFFICIENTS
AND DEGREE OF ASSOCIATED CONCOMITANT VARIANCE**

| r | $r^2$ | % of Common Variance |
|---|---|---|
| 1.00 | 1.00 | 100 |
| .90 | .81 | 81 |
| .80 | .64 | 64 |
| .70 | .49 | 49 |
| .60 | .36 | 36 |
| .50 | .25 | 25 |
| .40 | .16 | 16 |
| .30 | .09 | 9 |
| .20 | .04 | 4 |
| .10 | .01 | 1 |

correlational methods to the area of behavioral and physiological research, for when a given statistical relationship is known to exist between two variables, it is possible to predict the value of the second variable within a given range of accuracy, provided the value of the first variable is known.

Correlational techniques lend themselves well to the study of individual differences in motor learning. Through factor analysis (a statistical method requiring a complex series of correlational operations), it is possible to identify the few central factors which underlie performance on a wide variety of specific skills. Basic ability factors are identified through clusters of correlations in a matrix. When a number of specific skills show high correlation, it is assumed that there is a common factor or ability construct (strength, endurance, flexibility) which underlies the successful performance of all of these different tasks. Once identified, these common factors (ability constructs) represent behavioral traits or capacities which account for proficiency upon a variety of tasks. When an ability factor is operationally defined (e.g., a test score), it is possible, within given limits, to predict an individual's performance upon a criterion task which is dependent upon that ability. Subjects with high quantitative ability, for example, should acquire arithmetical skills with ease. In motor learning, individuals who possess high levels of manual dexterity should manifest a facility for learning to catch a ball which is either thrown or struck.

Correlational techniques have been applied successfully to the realm of testing itself, particularly in the areas of behavioral and applied physiological measurements. A primary requisite of any test is internal consistency or reliability. A test must first correlate with itself before it can rightly be employed to measure anything else. This internal consistency or reliability is reflected in the reliability coefficient, a correlation coefficient derived from the relationship between two repeated administrations of either the same test or alternate forms of the same test to the same group of subjects. The greater the tendency of every individual within the group to maintain his initial position in relation to the mean during the second administration of the test, the greater the reliability of the measure. The lower the reliability of a test, the greater the likelihood that the outcome is the result of chance.

A second and most critical application of correlational techniques to the area of testing relates to validity. Validity involves the correlation between some measure of behavioral or of physiological factors with a criterion measure of performance. The higher the validity coefficient, the greater the relationship between the factors comprising the initial measure and those comprising the criterion measure, hence, the greater the accuracy to predict ultimate performance from an initial baseline measure.

Although the statistical techniques thus far discussed are applicable only to conditions involving the treatment and interpretation of metric data, the physical educator is often confronted with situations involving frequency values in discrete categories—pass-fail grading or ordinal ranking, such as size place or order of finish in a race. Since frequency data does not lend itself to analysis through conventional statistical techniques, a number of nonparametric statistical methods have been developed which, while somewhat less accurate than parametric methods, manage to approximate their findings fairly closely. These nonparametric techniques enable the researcher to execute comparative as well as relational interpretations of frequency data.

### Nonparametric Statistics

A widely used method for comparison of frequency data is the chi-square technique of nonparametric statistical analysis. This method compares the observed number of cases falling in each category to the expected number, based upon the proportional representation of each subgroup in the entire population. A problem well suited to this form of analysis is if the acquisition of a given motor skill is contingent upon the sex of the learner. Are females more likely to acquire a given task than are males of equal ability? Assume that in a population comprised of 55 females and 45 males, 20 of the males and 35 of the females ultimately succeeded in acquiring the criterion task. This data can be expressed graphically in the form of a two-by-two contingency table by allowing the row headings to represent success or failure and the column headings to represent the sex of the subject.

|  | Females | Males | Totals* |
|---|---|---|---|
| Learned | 35 (30.25) | 20 (24.75) | 55 |
| Failed to learn | 20 (24.75) | 25 (20.25) | 45 |

---

*Note that row and column sums for the expected values equal those for the observed values.

The observed values are a given; the expected values (the parenthetical expressions) must be computed. The logic which underlies this computation is predicated upon the premise that if chance alone were operating, the percentage of members of either sex both passing and failing should be equal to the proportion of the entire population constituted by that group (males and females respectively, in this case). Since, in this example, the total population consists of 100 people, females constitute 55 percent while males constitute 45 percent. It is argued, therefore, that since females constitute 55 percent of the total population, they should also constitute 55 percent of all those who learn the task and 55 percent of all those who fail to do so. Since the total number of those learning was 55, the expected number of females learning is $(.55)(55) = 30.25$. Since the total number of those who did not learn was 45, the expected number of females who fail to learn is $(.55)(45) = 24.75$. It is further argued that since males constitute 45 percent of the total population, they should also constitute 45 percent of those learning and 45 percent of those who fail to learn. Since the total number of those learning was 55, the expected number of males learning is $(.45)(55) = 24.75$. Since the total number of those who did not learn was 45, the expected number of males who do not learn is $(.45)(45) = 20.25$. Upon examining the data, it becomes apparent that the rate of learning for females is higher than expected, that for males is lower. In contrast, the failure rate for females is lower than expected, that for males is higher. The ultimate question is if these differences between observed and expected values are merely the result of chance or if the learning of this particular task is actually contingent upon the sex of the learner.

The chi-square technique empirically enables the researcher to arrive at a conclusion concerning the likelihood of discrepancies between the observed and the expected values resulting from chance alone, and the magnitude of these differences serves as the test of the null hypothesis. The closer the observed values conform to the expected values, the greater the likelihood that the differences between these values are due to chance. The critical value necessary for rejecting a null hypothesis will vary according to the number of groups and the number of categories employed in the analysis.

In addition to statistical methods which allow for the comparative analysis of frequency data, there are techniques which can be employed to determine the degree of relationship between two sets of nonparametric data. If a researcher were interested in the degree of relationship between performance upon a reliable and valid objective measure of behavior (e.g., a test score) and a proficiency rating given by a panel of judges (e.g., a gymnastics or diving competition), product-moment correlation would not be applicable. By ranking subjects according to the judges' ratings ordinally and then ranking them again according to their test performance, it is possible to measure the degree of relationship between these two variables. This is accomplished through use of the rank correlation coefficient technique. This nonparametric statistical technique is based solely upon the ordinal rank of a score. If metric values are employed at all, they are used only as a basis for assessing ordinal ranks. The greater the agreement between each subject's respective standing (rank on each measure), the higher the correlation.

Statistical methods are valuable tools in assessing motor learning, but even the most sophisticated have limited application to practical situations. In a comparative study, for example, significant findings are indicative only of the fact that sufficient evidence exists to warrant the rejection of a null hypothesis; in no way do these findings constitute a direct proof of the hypothesis of the experiment. The fact that experimental groups differ in performance beyond the limits of chance does not conclusively prove that such differences are due to the experimental treatments received by those groups. A correlation coefficient expresses only the degree of linear relationship between two variables. This relationship in turn reflects the degree to which those variables share common factors. No correlational technique can be used to infer a causal relationship between any two variables: though two variables are strongly related in terms of common factors, the presence of the first is not necessarily the cause of the occurrence of the second. Even though all statistical methods provide accurate and concise techniques for treating and interpreting compilations of data, the most important factors in any research entail, first, selecting the appropriate method in the appropriate circumstance and, second, confining the conclusions to the limits of the statistical technique selected.

*Bibliography*

Baumgartner, T.A. and A.S. Jackson. *Measurement for Evaluation in Physical Education.* Boston: Houghton Mifflin Co., 1975.

Blalock, H.M. *Social Statistics.* New York: McGraw-Hill, 1960.

Dotson, C.O. and D.R. Kirkendall. *Statistics for Physical Education, Health and Recreation.* New York: Harper and Row, 1974.

Edwards, A.L. *Experimental Design in Psychological Research.* New York: Holt, Rinehart and Winston, 1972.

———. *Statistical Methods.* 3rd ed. New York: Holt, Rinehart and Winston, 1973.

Guilford, J.P. and B. Fruchter. *Fundamental Statistics in Psychology and Education.* 6th ed. New York: McGraw-Hill, 1977.

Minium, E.W. *Statistical Reasoning in Psychology and Education.* New York: John Wiley, 1978.

Popham, W.J. and K.A. Sirotnik. *Educational Statistics: Use and Interpretation.* 2nd ed. New York: Harper and Row, 1973.

Thorndike, R.L. and E.P. Hagen. *Measurement and Evaluation in Psychology and Education.* 4th ed. New York: John Wiley, 1977.

# CHAPTER 4

# *Transfer of Learning*

THE CONCEPT OF TRANSFER is central to the learning and performance of verbal as well as motor activities. It provides the individual with knowledge and skills which may be readily applied beyond the confines of the classroom. Despite this fundamental influence of transfer upon all forms of learning, its role in the acquisition of motor skills differs from its role in the learning and performance of verbal behavior. Although the acquisition of complex motor activities embodies conceptual or ideational elements directed to the principles, goals, and objectives of the activity, as well as motoric factors which are solely confined to executing the precise neuromuscular responses peculiar to the task, the ideational elements are highly verbal in nature and therefore much broader in scope than are the motoric elements.

As has been mentioned, a prior knowledge of the principles of softball may facilitate the understanding of the rules and strategies of baseball, but the prior acquisition of specific softball skills, such as throwing, catching, and hitting, may interfere with the acquisition of these same skills when they are employed in baseball. Such interference results from differences in the size and weight of the equipment and in the timing of the movements used in each game. Although a prime objective of coaching is to develop a player's ability to transfer skills acquired during the practice session to the actual game situation, and although the physical educator clearly strives to teach activities that will have carry-over value to later life, the highly specific nature of motor skills virtually precludes predicting the precise degree to which the acquisition of a given motor skill will be facilitated or inhibited by the prior acquisition of related skills.

The contingency of transfer of learning upon the presence of identical elements in the initial and transfer tasks or instead upon the application of broad general principles common to both tasks is a subject of major controversy. Regardless to which theoretical position one adheres, the presence of nonidentical yet highly similar elements within the two tasks confounds the study of transfer of learning. In the case of the identical elements theory, it is the degree of physical similarity (the size, shape, or weight of the equipment as well as the movement patterns) between the two tasks which is believed to result in interference. In the case of the general principles theory, however, interference is believed to result from the degree of conceptual similarity (the rules, strategies, and procedures) employed in the execution of the two tasks. The area of transfer has been the subject of intensive theoretical speculation and experimental study, and its practical ramifications in the acquisition of motor skills bear critically upon the sequence employed in the teaching of such skills.

There are two fundamental considerations which underlie all transfer of learning: the type of transfer, which can be either positive, negative, or neutral; and the direction of transfer, which can be either proactive or retroactive. Reduced to simplest terms, the basic issue of transfer of learning pertains to how the acquisition of a particular skill is affected by prior experience (proaction) or the interpolation of a different activity during the course of acquisition (retroaction). If the learning of a motor skill, riding a bicycle let us say, is facilitated by the prior experience of having ridden a tricycle, then a positive transfer of learning is said to exist between these two skills. If, on the other hand, learning to ride a bicycle is made more difficult, or inhibited, by the prior experience of tricycle riding, a negative transfer is said to exist between the two skills. If the learning of an initial skill apparently has neither a positive nor a negative effect upon the acquisition of a succeeding skill, transfer is said to be neutral.

### Retroaction and Proaction

Research upon transfer of learning has centered on the use of two basic experimental designs, the proactive and the retroactive paradigms. The design for proaction involves the effects of a previously acquired task upon the acquisition of a succeeding skill. The simplest form of the proactive design compares the performance of an experimental group which receives instruction on an initial task (the independent variable) with a control group receiving no such instruction, using some criterion measure or transfer task (the dependent variable). If the experimental group demonstrates performance that is significantly superior to that of the control group, a positive transfer exists between the initial task and the criterion task. This positive transfer is referred to as proactive facilitation. If, in contrast, the experimental group is significantly inferior to the control group upon the criterion task, then negative transfer or proactive inhibition has occurred.

The basic paradigm for retroaction allows initial acquisition of the criterion task by both groups, the experimental and the control. The experimental group is then taught a second task (the independent variable) while the control group remains inactive. Both groups are then retested on the initial skill (the dependent variable). If the experimental group's performance is significantly superior to that of the control group, retroactive facilitation is said to have occurred. But should the experimental group's performance be significantly poorer than that of the control group, retroactive inhibition results. (See Figure 4-1)

**Figure 4-1**

**SUMMARY OF SEVERAL TRANSFER DESIGNS**

| Design | Group | | Original Task | Transfer Task |
|:---:|---|---|---|---|
| 1 | Experimental | | Learn A | Learn B |
| | Control | | (Rests) | Learn B |
| 2 | Experimental | Pretest on $B^1$ | Learn A | Learn B |
| | Control | Pretest on $B^1$ | (Rests) | Learn B |
| 3 | Experimental | | Learn A | Learn B |
| | Control | | Learn B | Learn A |
| 4 | Experimental | | Learn A | Learn $B_1$ |
| | Control | | Learn A | Learn B |
| 5 | Experimental and Control | | Learn A | Learn B |

Although a number of theoretical explanations have been offered to account for the phenomena of retroaction and proaction, none provides an entirely satisfactory explanation. Theoretical controversies over the nature of negative transfer have characteristically revolved around two fundamental issues: the role of retention and that of interference. Proponents of a retention hypothesis contend that negative transfer results from the weakening or decay of the initial response over time alone (forgetting); those of an interference hypothesis, that the acquisition of a second response creates competition with the original one for the available storage capacity (memory). Since the demands of the situation outweigh the capacity of the learner, there is a resultant decrement in performance.

A classical explanation for the phenomenon of retroactive inhibition is found in the preservation hypothesis, which proposes that the learning process continues for a brief period after the cessation of actual practice. It is argued that the interpolation of different activities interferes with this "after-image" of the original learning and results in interference, inhibition, and negative transfer when the original activity is resumed. Although this theory appears superficially sound, McGeoch and Irion (1961) identify several inherent contradictions in its logic which seriously undermine its viability.

The first objection to the preservation theory as a valid explanation of retroactive inhibition is based upon the premise that the actual preservation phenomenon is a short-term process. Although preservation is believed to exist only for a few moments following the cessation of practice upon the initial activity, the interpolation of additional activities hours and even days after the cessation of this initial practice resulted in interference, inhibition, and negative transfer when performance upon the original task was resumed. These findings seem to indicate that retroactive inhibition is the result of factors other than interference with the process of preservation.

A second objection is based upon the argument that, if the preservation theory were indeed correct, the amount of interference associated with an interpolated activity should be directly proportional to the intensity of the activity. If interference with the processes of preservation were, in fact, the causal element in retroactive inhibition, then, clearly, more intense activities should result in greater interference than would activities of lesser intensity. Unfortunately, research evidence has failed to corroborate this contention. The intensity of the interpolated activity and the degree of resultant retroactive inhibition are apparently independent factors.

A third critical objection to the preservation theory is predicated upon the similarity between the initial and the interpolated activities. According to the preservation hypothesis, the interpolation of activities highly similar to the initial activities should exert a far lesser degree of interference upon the preservation process as compared to the degree of interference that would result from the interpolation of highly dissimilar activities. The preponderance of the evidence, however, indicates that the greatest degree of negative transfer tends to occur when the initial and interpolated activities manifest high similarity. If the preservation hypothesis were indeed viable, practice upon a highly similar task would clearly facilitate rather than inhibit performance upon the initial task.

The fourth and most decisive argument against the preservation theory is that it can only be applied to the retroactive paradigm. Since the preservation hypothesis is wholly untenable in situations involving proactive inhibition, preservation theory in and of itself cannot be regarded as a valid explanation of the entire phenomenon of transfer of learning.

In view of the shortcomings of the preservation hypothesis, McGeoch and Irion have proposed a two-factor theory of retroactive inhibition to account for time and interference. According to this theory, increasing amounts of the original response become unlearned (forgotten) as a consequence of time alone, while the remaining original responses are simultaneously subjected to competition (interference) from the interpolated activity (new task). This theory provides a reasonably logical explanation of retroactive inhibition. The theoretical basis of proaction has yet to be discussed.

Although the effects of proactive inhibition have great bearing upon practical learning situations in terms of the degree to which prior experience will affect current learning, the bulk of theoretical research upon transfer has, until fairly recently, been overwhelmingly concerned with retroaction, particularly as it occurs under highly controlled laboratory conditions. Current theoretical explanations of proaction are therefore primarily derived from prior findings concerned with retroaction. It is generally conceded that proaction results from the effects of competition only; retroaction adds the factor of time.

Further support for the interference hypothesis is provided by Hicks and Cohn (1975), who write that the amount of retroactive inhibition has been found to be an increasing function of the amount of interpolated learning in the case of verbal as well as motor tasks. In contrast to the predictions of the two-factor theory of retroactive inhibition, no change in the effects of interpolated learning was observed as the length of the retention interval was increased. The authors also failed to observe any evidence of proactive inhibition, and conclude, therefore, that in terms of the particular motor tasks employed in this investigation (the Tsai-Partington numbers test), retroaction and proaction do not appear to be the result of a common interference mechanism. Based upon the lack of observed interaction between the number of interpolated learning trials and the length of the retention interval, Hicks and Cohn contend that the interference processes operating in the case of motor skill acquisition differ from those which affect verbal learning.

Dickinson and Higgins (1977), in contrast, observed proactive and retroactive interference effects in the case of a linear arm-positioning task. These interference effects diminished, however, as the movement characteristics (length of movement, in this case) of the criterion response were altered. The authors hold that these findings lend support to the contention that the acquisition and retention of verbal and motor skills are prone to interference from either prior or interpolated activities with characteristics similar to the criterion response.

*Response Generalization and Task Similarity*

The acquisition and performance of any motor task is dependent upon the elicitation of the appropriate sequence of responses by given stimuli. These stimuli include verbal commands, lights, sounds, or the mere presence of specialized equipment or apparatus, such as a "universal gym" or a basket and backboard. The precise relationship between given stimuli and a particular pattern of responses is defined by the nature of the criterion task and constitutes a critical theoretical factor in the transfer of learning. In essence, the degree to which intertask transfer will be positive or negative is largely dependent upon the respective stimulus-response relationships governing the acquisition and performance of both tasks. The level of proficiency with which the criterion task is performed is taken as an operational measure of the correctness of the response.

According to Deese (1958), the degree of positive transfer between two tasks (responses) is related to the degree of compatibility between them. The greater the number of elements common to both tasks, the greater the transfer from one to the other. Learning algebra will be greatly facilitated by the prior acquisition of basic arithmetic skills since both arithmetical and algebraic operations rely upon common principles. In contrast, responses which are mutually exclusive (eliciting one precludes the possibility of simultaneously eliciting the second, as in sleep and wakefulness) and opposing (e.g., running and sitting) are most prone to interfere with one other. This interference results in negative transfer, particularly when the responses are elicited under identical stimulus conditions.

Assume that there are two groups of individuals, and that subjects in the first group have been trained to run at the sound of a starting gun while those in the second group have received no such training. Suppose that after a suitable training interval, the experimenter decides that all subjects in both groups will now be taught to sit at the sound of the gun. Obviously, in this case, the subjects in the second group should have far less difficulty mastering the criterion task than those in the first group, who had received training on an opposing task performed under identical conditions.

Deese contends that tasks which are highly compatible and tend to flow along some form of continuum (sprinting, running, trotting, jogging, fast walking) are, in contrast to mutually exclusive responses, likely to transfer positively in an identical stimulus situation. Assume that the preceding hypothetical experiment were to be repeated but that this time the first group of subjects was initially trained to jog at the sound of the starting gun. Following a suitable training interval, the group was to be retrained and required to walk quickly when presented with the same starting signal employed initially to elicit the jogging response. According to Deese, there should be less negative transfer in this situation.

Gagné et al. (1950) write that the critical element in determining transfer of learning pertains to the degree of intratask similarity governing the relationships among the stimulus and response elements within a given task. The authors contend that this similarity may be varied in four ways: by making the stimulus elements in the second task more like those in the first task; by making the stimulus elements in the second task less like those of the first; by altering each of the stimuli in the second task along a scale of similarity with those of the first; and by reversing the relationships between the stimuli and responses in the second task. The first three variations tend to result in positive transfer, and the fourth in negative transfer. Gagné's contention is supported by empirical evidence which indicates that general ability factors decline in importance as proficiency develops, i.e., the higher the level of performance, the more task-specific the underlying factors become. (See Chapter 7 for a discussion of the role of abilities in motor learning.)

These transfer effects are believed to result from a generalization gradient which affects both stimulus and response elements. Gagné suggests that these gradients, which themselves are mediated by cognitive processes, exert their greatest effects upon transfer during the initial phases of skill acquisition, but diminish in importance as proficiency is attained and the required discriminations become more firmly established. The concept of the *stimulus* generalization gradient is based upon the assumption that the acquisition of a given response to a particular stimulus situation will increase the chances of making the same response when one is confronted with a stimulus similar to the original one. Thus, an individual taught to stop at a red light will readily transfer this response to a situation in which he is presented with an orange light.

The authors further state that the processes which underlie transfer of learning are also dependent upon a *response* generalization gradient. This position is based upon the assumption that an individual who learns a specific response to a given stimulus also acquires the tendency to make different responses to the same stimulus. A person taught to perform a task in a specific fashion often develops alternative styles of executing the same task. Someone who has learned to serve a tennis ball in a particular manner may vary his performance to attain greater comfort or efficiency. These tendencies to generalize a response decrease, however, as the similarity between the initial response and the transfer task decrease. Gagné et al. write that although a motor response is believed to vary in terms of such aspects as its direction, distance, force, and rate, the degree of similarity between any two motor responses is assessed in terms of the actual results of the movement rather than the patterns of muscular activity employed in the execution of the response. Two movements are viewed as similar when they both fulfill a similar environmental goal (e.g., an overhand throw and a side arm throw). An individual who is taught to throw overhand may also tend to accomplish the stated environmental goal by throwing side arm.

*Similarity and Negative Transfer.* Dey (1977) writes that the relationship between similarity and negative transfer rests largely in the concept of the stimulus-response generalization gradient. Two hypotheses based upon this concept have been formulated, but so far they have been applied mainly to verbal learning. The first of these is the hypothesis of parasitic reinforcement, which states that reinforced practice during the acquisition of the initial task strengthens not only that particular response but similar responses as well, thereby increasing the chance of negative transfer. The second hypothesis is based upon the concept of a mediational chain which enables an entire response pattern to occur in a programed sequence. The greater the degree of similarity between the correct elements in the sequence and other extraneous responses which are readily available (e.g., stepping sideward instead of forward during the delivery in bowling), the greater the chance of obtaining negative transfer. In both hypotheses, the greater the similarity between the stimulus situations of the initial and transfer tasks (similarities in the type of equipment employed, method of instruction, or surrounding conditions) and the greater the similarity between the response requirements of the initial task and the transfer task (stepping forward with the right leg in the first task, as opposed to stepping forward with the left leg in the second), the greater the resultant stimulus-response generalization gradient and the greater the likelihood of negative transfer resulting between the tasks.

Dey observed significant interaction effects between stimulus similarity, response similarity, and negative transfer in the acquisition of a motor task (card sorting). These interactions were attributed to the tendency of a given motor response to deviate from its correct course because of conflict with other responses. The author contends that a given stimulus invokes not only its own response but also elicits responses which have been previously conditioned to similar stimuli. A gymnastics student who learns the handspring following the prior acquisition of the neckspring may often confuse the two responses. The execution of the handspring will result in the presence of responses, such as bending the elbows, appropriate to the neckspring. The conflict between these two simultaneously evoked, incompatible responses results in the emergence of a conflict resultant or hybrid response (which is neither a handspring nor a neckspring) lying somewhere between the two conflicting responses. Dey proposes that the amount of negative transfer and interference are directly proportional to the distance (as measured along a continuum of similarity) between the correct response and the hybrid one. The distance (degree of similarity) between these two responses (correct and hybrid) is believed to increase in proportion to the distance between the correct response (the handspring, in this case) and the erroneous one (the neckspring).

An example of a verbal conflict resultant is the language student whose prior knowledge of Spanish interferes with his learning of French. He learns the correct response, the French word for window (la fenêtre), confuses it with an incorrect response, the Spanish word for window (la ventana), and comes up with a hybrid response, the nonsense word "la fentana." The greater the similarity (distance) between the French word and the Spanish one, the greater the likelihood of confusing the two and, even more important, the more difficult it becomes to distinguish between the hybrid response and the correct one.

Dey summarized by saying that an inverse relationship should exist between interference and response similarity.* He argues that the greater the similarity between the correct response and the conflict resultant, the greater the strength of the hybrid response in relation to that of the correct response, and the greater the resultant interference. Developing a "bad habit" in the performance of a motor skill constitutes a common example of the effects of such interference. The greater the similarity in the prevailing stimulus conditions (a tennis court and a badminton court), the greater the likelihood of eliciting an incorrect response (a tennis swing while playing badminton or a badminton strike while playing tennis). The greater the similarity between the two responses (the tennis stroke and the badminton stroke, in this case), the more difficult it is to distinguish between the hybrid response (either a tennis stroke which partially resembles a badminton stroke or a badminton stroke which resembles a tennis stroke) and the correct response (either the proper tennis swing or the proper badminton swing). Finally, the greater the resemblance between the correct response and the hybrid response, the more subtle the decrement in performance, and the greater the

---

*The more two motor responses are alike, the greater the negative transfer and, conversely, the less the similarity, the less the negative transfer.

difficulty in detecting it and effecting the appropriate corrections. Gross mistakes are far easier to detect and correct than are subtle errors.

## Figure 4-2

## HYPOTHETICAL TRANSFER SURFACE *

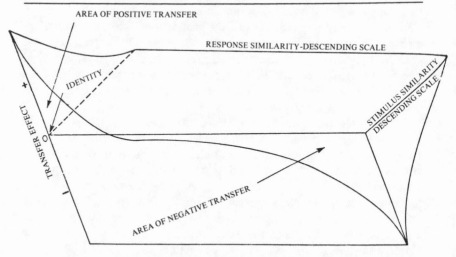

\* The amount of transfer (positive and negative) as a joint function of stimulus similarity and response similarity.

Osgood (1949) postulates three general principles of transfer which are represented in the form of a topological surface. (See Figure 4-2) The first principle states that positive transfer between two learning tasks will increase in proportion to the degree of stimulus similarity, provided that the responses are identical in both situations. The second states that if the stimuli are identical in both tasks but the responses are different, negative transfer directly proportional to the degree of dissimilarity between the responses results. The third principle states that in cases where the stimuli and the responses are different for each respective task, negative transfer ensues and increases as the degree of similarity between the two respective stimuli increases. In essence (although it appears paradoxical), according to Osgood, when one is learning two tasks requiring dissimilar responses, the greater the similarity between stimuli, the greater the resultant interference, negative transfer, and inhibition. It is due precisely to this last factor that transfer between motor tasks (all of which are largely comprised of highly specific responses) is characteristically negative.

Relating Osgood's theoretical model to practical problems in motor learning, one can see that a critical factor affecting transfer is the nature of the learning situation itself. Generally speaking, positive transfer will result if the learner is required to make the identical response in both situations, provided there is some degree of similarity between the two. A child enrolled in a class in bicycle safety, for example, should manifest a high degree of positive transfer when learning to stop at a blinking red light after first having learned the response of stopping for a steady red light. The degree of similarity between the two stimuli is high and the response in both cases is identical. In contrast, negative transfer results when the stimulus situation remains the same but the response must be changed, as in the case of a cyclist who changes from a bicycle with coaster brakes to one with hand brakes. The stimuli that elicit the response of stopping are the same in both cases, but the actual nature of the response is different. Another example of a negative transfer situation is the baseball player who must swing at a pitch when the coach kicks the dirt with his left foot but must "take" the pitch if the coach steps forward with the same foot.

Although Osgood's model has furthered the understanding of the processes which underlie transfer of learning, its primary focus is upon the degree of similarity between the stimulus and response situations which prevail during the elicitation and performance of the initial and the criterion learning tasks. Holding (1976) finds the degree of such similarity far less important in determining the amount and direction of transfer than certain critical factors related to the conditions of training, the characteristics of the subjects, and the nature of the experimental tasks. These factors include the ability level of the subjects, their level of mastery of the initial task, the amount of information feedback provided during the acquisition of the initial and criterion tasks, and the nature and complexity of these tasks.

Holding argues that positive and negative transfer are relative rather than absolute values since, to a varying degree, both are present in every transfer of learning situation. He contends that the perceived consequences of transfer (either positive or negative) are often due to methodological or procedural factors (e.g., the use of a particular scoring system), rather than factors inherent in the initial or the criterion learning task. Negative transfer is viewed as a situation in which positive transfer is misplaced. According to Holding, a subject trained to behave in a certain way will, under similar circumstances, continue to do so. When maintenance of the initial behavior is viewed as correct by the teacher or experimenter, positive transfer results. But if the initial behavior is incorrect, negative transfer ensues. In essence, negative transfer results when the criterion has been changed but the subject's behavior has not.

There are a number of factors which contribute to such negative transfer. The less skilled an individual, the greater the likelihood of negative transfer when confronted with a similar yet different response situation. For example, the would-be "do-it-yourselfer" with limited experience in wiring a doorbell causes extensive damage when he attempts repairs upon a complex electrical circuit. Negative transfer may also result from a lack of information about how to discriminate between two tasks. Even though situations are different, the learner may not have sufficient information to know how they differ. When the learning task itself does not provide sufficient information to allow the subject to discriminate, such information must be provided in the form of advanced instruction on the specific properties of the learning tasks. Unfortunately, the failure to remember such instructions often results in negative transfer.

The subject's ability to differentiate accurately between the requirements of the initial task and those of the criterion task is implicit in the nature of learning transfer. The failure to make this discrimination results in negative transfer and is a consequence of one of two fundamentally opposing factors: the high degree of cognitive involvement in the initial task with the accompanying broad patterns of response generalization, and overlearning of the initial task. If the first factor is in operation, an individual who has attained a minimal degree of skill at serving a tennis ball will more than likely apply the same response pattern trying to execute a badminton serve. Although there is a great deal of conceptual similarity between these two responses, they differ considerably in terms of the speed and force of the movement and the mass of the striking implement. Therefore, generalizing the principles which govern the performance of the initial task to the execution of the transfer task is an incorrect response and results in negative transfer. The second factor applies sequentially: the better learned a task, the more automatic its execution; hence, the greater the likelihood that the subject will reproduce that response even when the prevailing circumstances have been altered.

It would appear from the preceding discussion that, regardless of the extent of prior experience, negative transfer must always result when a second task which is similar to the first is acquired. As previously stated, however, almost all transfer of learning involves positive as well as negative elements. Often the ultimate factor which determines the nature of transfer in a given situation stems from the environmental consequences of the activity.

Assume that an individual who has initially learned to drive an automobile with an automatic transmission is later taught to drive a standard transmission vehicle. The progress of this individual is compared to that of a second subject with no prior driving experience who is taught standard shift initially. If the person with the prior knowledge of driving experiences only minor difficulties (the car bucks or stalls) and is able to apply his previously acquired driving skill to the new situation, it can be said that a positive transfer exists between the two tasks. If, however, after a suitable training period, both drivers are faced with an unexpected situation and the one with prior experience commits an error (improper synchronization of the clutch with the accelerator) resulting in a loss of control of the vehicle, the logical conclusion is that negative transfer has resulted. Frequently, the outcome of the behavior determines if transfer is positive or negative.

### Defining the Criterion

The problems in an objective investigation of transfer of learning are compounded not only by variations in the learning situation, but by ambiguity in the definition of learning itself. Although a number of theoretical definitions are largely accepted, only in the experimental context is learning operationally defined. Operational definitions range over a broad spectrum of behavioral objectives, but several particular examples tend to predominate.

A common approach dichotomizes the acquisition process, viewing the criterion response as wholly learned or wholly unlearned. While such a method can greatly facilitate the objective estimation of learning rate, it fails to account for variations in the quality of performance following the initial acquisition of the criterion task. A typical application of the dichotomous approach is to record the number of attempts required by an individual to perform a headstand successfully for the first time. Although this procedure provides an objective index of learning rate (the number of trials required to acquire the skill), it cannot account for variations in performance as higher levels of proficiency are attained. An example of the application of dichotomous scoring to the measurement of behavior is pass-fail grading (e.g., the evaluation of performance upon the Kraus-Weber test).

An alternative approach to operationally defining learning uses a dichotomized variable in which some criterion measure of proficiency, such as time or score, is dichotomized. Thus, a given point in the distribution is designated as the cutoff point for success or failure. Running 100 yards in ten seconds or less, scoring 75 percent or better on a given number of foul shots, or bowling five consecutive closed frames illustrate the operational definition of learning based upon dichotomized continuous variables.

Still another approach employs actual continuous variables, such as time, score, or distance. In such a situation, the researcher views learning as an infinitely variable phenomenon in which all gradations of performance are possible. Examples are found in many varied situations: the time elapsed to run a set distance; the actual number of baskets scored in a game; the number of pull-ups or push-ups completed; the time, height, or distance covered in a jump or throw; or the score achieved on a test.

Added to the problem of defining learning in either dichotomous or continuous terms is the choice of level of proficiency demanded by the researcher from his subjects. Studies which operationally define learning in terms of the initial acquisition of a task are dealing with very different ability factors from those concerned with the attainment of high levels of proficiency.

Fitts (1964) postulates a three-stage model of skill acquisition (see Chapter 2). According to Fitts, since insight and understanding are critical factors in early learning, the initial acquisition of a skill is heavily dependent upon cognition and associated verbal abilities. These initial stages of motor learning are characterized as well by a high degree of conscious mediation in the regulation and control of movement. The second stage of learning involves a transition from cognitive or ideational factors to kinesthetic or proprioceptive ones. "Having the idea" of the skill no longer suffices, for at this point in the learning process the learner must come to task with the situation and learn to make the appropriate adjustments and regulations in response to changes in pressure, force, and direction. The ideational knowledge acquired through explanation and demonstration during the first stage must be translated into performance in the second. The third stage of skill acquisition involves relegating the control processes governing the performance of a motor task to lower centers of the nervous system. When this is accomplished, the execution and associated adjustments of the task are effected at subconscious levels.

That clear differences exist between the requisite ability factors in the early phases of motor learning and those during the later stages is strengthened by the work of Fleishman and Rich (1963). Their findings indicate that early learning is critically dependent upon visual abilities, advanced levels upon proprioceptive abilities. Relating the work of Fleishman and Rich to transfer in motor learning, it is apparent that the findings of transfer studies predicated upon the early stages of skill acquisition have little application to the attainment of high levels of proficiency.

Hinrichs (1970) provides experimental evidence in support of the findings of Fleishman and Rich and Fitts by observing that the abilities required in the performance of a motor task change during the course of learning. These changes occur in a relatively systematic fashion from one stage of practice to the next, the abilities stabilizing as the final level of proficiency is attained. Hinrichs observed that the proportion of task-specific variance (the elements unique to a given task, e.g., the timing of precise patterns of muscular force) increases as proficiency is developed and the proportion of nonspecific variance (elements related to concepts, methods, and strategies) decreases. Since the achievement of high levels of proficiency in a skill is dependent upon factors distinct from those which underlie its initial acquisition, any study dealing with transfer of learning must require the subjects to demonstrate equal levels of proficiency upon the initial and transfer tasks.

### Task Complexity

Research upon transfer of learning is also complicated by differences in the complexity of the tasks. According to Day (1956), difficulty is measured in terms of such relative factors as the speed and complexity of the response. The speed of a task is a reciprocal function of the time in which that task must be performed (the greater its speed, the less the available response time). The complexity of a task embodies such factors as the order or sequence in which the constituent elements must be executed (the more complicated the sequence, the more difficult the task), the number of elements in the sequence (the more responses required, the greater the difficulty), and the level of precision required (as the level of precision of the response is increased, the margin for error is correspondingly decreased). It appears obvious that the prior acquisition of a difficult task should facilitate the acquisition of a simpler one (positive transfer), but Holding (1962) writes that there is no conclusive evidence supporting positive transfer between a difficult and an easy task to be greater than between an easy and a difficult one.

Holding contends that since task difficulty is relative rather than absolute, the key factor governing transfer between tasks of different levels of complexity is the principle of inclusion. When two similar tasks of different complexity are comprised of physically identical elements, the simpler task will share all of its elements with the more complex; the latter will contain additional elements. Riding a single-speed bicycle equipped with coaster brakes involves elements of balance, timing, and coordination; riding a ten-speed bicycle requires all of these plus the cognitive aspect associated with the decisions involved in shifting gears. If the more complex task is acquired initially, the acquisition of the simpler task should be facilitated since its elements are included in the first task. If, however, the task emphasizes principles governing broad response tendencies (anticipation or accuracy), as opposed to specific movement characteristics (force or speed), transfer will usually proceed from the easier to the more complex since the simpler task includes the concepts and methods that are applicable to the more complex activity.

Of all the elements contributing to the complexity of a task, speed has been the focus of greatest concern. Ammons et al. (1956) observed that in the case of a pursuit-rotor tracking* task, an overall inverse relationship was observed between speed and performance: the faster the pacing of the task, the more poorly all subjects performed, regardless of prior training. When the rate of the final (criterion) task was equal to or lower than that of the training (initial) task, the amount of transfer was directly proportional to the similarity between the rates of the two tasks. When the speed requirements of the final task were very high, however, there were no significant differences in performance as reflected by time on target score, regardless of the speed of their initial learning. Similar findings were obtained by Baker et al. (1950) for performance upon a tracking task. The authors observed that the greatest amount of transfer resulted when the speed of the final and initial tasks did not differ. When differences did exist, however, the amount of transfer was greater when the initial task had the higher speed.

Jensen (1976) studied the effects of variations in speed and complexity (tracking pattern) of a task upon transfer, and observed that, regardless of the tracking pattern, subjects who initially practiced at speeds most similar to the criterion speed performed most effectively. Conversely, the greater the difference between the speed of the training task and that of the criterion task, the poorer the performance. Jensen writes that although the study failed to yield conclusive findings on the interaction between initial training speed and task difficulty, such effects tend to be most conspicuous during early learning and diminish during the course of practice. Initial training is most effective when carried out at a speed identical to that of the criterion task. While a slightly slower training speed may yield acceptable criterion performance, very slow training will be detrimental.

Sage and Hornak (1978) employed a pursuit-rotor tracking task and observed no significant differences in transfer between the performance of one group practicing at the criterion speed throughout training and that of a second group practicing under conditions of gradual and progressive increments in speed. The authors contend that transfer scores of subjects trained by different methods will not differ

---

*In pursuit-rotor tracking, a handheld stylus is kept in contact with a fixed point on a rotating turntable whose speed can be varied by the experimenter.

significantly as the speed of pretransfer training approaches that of the criterion task.

Boswell and Irion (1975) observed asymmetrical transfer between similar learning tasks which vary in difficulty. The authors used a pursuit-rotor tracking task and varied the speed of initial training and criterion performance conditions. The resultant transfer when the training (initial) speed was somewhat lower than the criterion speed was greater than that obtained when the speed of the training task was slightly higher than the criterion speed. The authors hold that these findings were due to greater learning at the lower initial speed, which was reflected in superior performance at the criterion speed. They conclude that the duration of the initial training period is critical in learning and must be considered along with speed and difficulty.

Similar findings were obtained by Rivenes and Caplan (1972), who observed greater transfer when the initial speed was less than the criterion speed on a pursuit-rotor tracking task. Livesey and Laszlo (1979) contend that much of the disagreement on the effects of variations in speed and task complexity on transfer results from the failure to differentiate between the perceived goal of the learner in the initial task and in the transfer task. The authors argue that the main element in transfer is the degree to which common strategies are employed in the execution of both tasks. The identification of these strategies will result in more reliable prediction of the direction and amount of transfer.

A major consideration in the study of transfer of learning pertains to the nature of the criterion task itself. Researchers frequently select tasks that are low in complexity, such as pursuit-rotor tracking, card sorting, and finger maze tracing, because performance upon such skills readily lends itself to objective analysis. Since transfer studies have focused primarily upon the broad underlying theoretical mechanisms governing the transfer of concepts and ideas rather than upon the acquisition of the criterion skills as an end in itself, relatively little attention has been given to the role of such task-related factors as speed, complexity, and redundancy in transfer of motor skill. The relevance of findings based on simple tasks and emphasizing the transfer of ideational elements to complex learning situations which stress task-specific elements* is of questionable validity.

### Verbal-Motor Transfer

Transfer between the ideational elements and the specific temporal and spatial aspects of skill acquisition is a major area of theoretical

---

*Temporal and spatial patterning and the modulation of muscular force.

inquiry for the researcher and the physical educator alike. In essence, to what extent does a knowledge of the principles required in the execution of the task, or an insight into and understanding of its overall purposiveness, actually facilitate its acquisition? Although a number of studies have been conducted in this area, the findings are by no means conclusive. Davies (1972) found that while the learning curves were similar for two groups of beginning archery students, the group receiving verbal tuition acquired the skill more rapidly and performed in a manner more consistently superior throughout the study. Mohr and Barrett (1972) were concerned with the effects of the knowledge of mechanical principles upon the acquisition of intermediate swimming skills. Students who were taught the mechanical principles governing efficient swimming techniques performed significantly better on tests of form and power than students who received standard instruction.

The question of transfer from verbal to motor learning is compounded by a number of related factors. A critical element in limiting the amount of transfer from ideational to motoric activities is the factor structure of the criterion task itself. According to Cratty (1973), the more adequately a motor task can be verbally described, the greater the likelihood that the amount of transfer resulting from a verbal learning situation to a motor task is contingent upon the complexity of the task and the degree of latitude permitted when defining the criteria of learning.

In the case of a simple motor skill such as bar pressing, a large segment of the skill's factor structure is readily accounted for by the set of verbal instructions stipulating that the learner press the bar. In the case of a complex motor activity, such as executing a gymnastic routine, verbal instruction accounts for an extremely limited segment of the factor structure. As the complexity of the task increases, verbal descriptions become virtually ineffectual as a mechanism for communicating the intricacies of the activity. Success in these highly complex motor activities is contingent upon precise, rapid, kinesthetic regulation rather than upon ideation. An individual can be subjected to intensive verbal instruction in the techniques of gymnastics, and yet have no more success in their actual execution than an equally able individual who received no such prior instruction.

Irion (1966) proposed that the complexity of any motor learning situation can be viewed in terms of availability of the response and selectivity of the task. A learning situation in which high response availability is coupled with low task selectivity is extremely simple; almost any response the learner is capable of eliciting will suffice to execute the task correctly (e.g., flicking a switch). It is precisely this type of learning situation that is most prone to positive transfer from verbal learning to motor learning. The selectivity of the task is so low that it allows the broadest possible latitude of responses which can be perceived as correct—it becomes exceedingly difficult to "miss." Conversely, tasks in which low response availability is coupled with high task selectivity reflect little if any positive transfer from verbal to motor learning. These tasks call for extremely precise responses that involve temporal and spatial rather than ideational factors. In such highly complex tasks (competitive diving, gymnastics, or figure skating), there is virtually no margin of error latitude. Merely having the "right idea" of what is required no longer suffices as evidence of learning.

It becomes ever more apparent that the extent of positive transfer between ideational and motor learning diminishes as the kinesthetic complexity of the motor task increases. According to Granit (1970), the attainment of high levels of motoric proficiency is a function of an individual's capacity to deal with real differences in the temporal and spatial displacements and accelerations of the body segments rather than of his capacity to process and abstract verbal information. Simply stated, an individual may have a perfect idea of what is required in the execution of a skill but at the same time be wholly incapable of performing it with any acceptable degree of proficiency. Although cognition and ideation are important in the initial stages of motor learning, high levels of proficiency are attained when the appropriate segments of the body are in the correct position, exerting the precise amount of force at the exact instant in time.

It should be clearly evident that any transfer between verbal and motor learning will be confined either to extremely simple tasks, to tasks in which high levels of proficiency are not required, or to the earliest stages in the acquisition of complex physical activities. This proposition is confirmed by Deese (1958), who writes that when the motoric aspect of a skill is relatively uncomplex, verbal pretraining yields great positive transfer. If the motoric aspects are highly complex, however, there is little or no transfer between verbal pretraining and the criterion task.

Since the learning criteria employed by Davies and by Mohr and Barrett provided a sizeable degree of latitude in the level of proficiency demanded of the subject, ideational factors clearly played a central role in the acquisition of the criterion tasks. Had the researchers demanded a higher level of proficiency, skill comparable to that of competitive-level performers, the prior verbal instruction would most likely have proven of little consequence in determining the ultimate degree of learning.

*Specific Versus Nonspecific Transfer*

The problem of task-to-task transfer is central to the development of proficiency during the later stages of motor learning. The theoretical basis of task-to-task transfer is contingent upon the presence of relatively broad behavioral traits or abilities in the learner that tend to support performance on a variety of tasks. Fleishman (1967) defines an ability as a capacity for processing certain types of information. The successful acquisition of such fundamental arithmetical skills as addition, subtraction, multiplication, and division depends upon the degree of quantitative ability possessed by the learner, despite the fact that each entails specific operations. The greater the degree of communality (in speed or strength or muscular endurance) between two tasks, the greater the probability of positive transfer between them. In the case of motor learning, transfer is particularly dependent upon common ability factors because every motor task is comprised of a highly specific series of elements or subtasks, ordered in a precise temporal and spatial pattern unique to a given skill. It is precisely this high degree of task specificity which severely limits transfer between even highly similar motor skills.

Since the acquisition of motor skill requires extrinsic or nonspecific factors (e.g., insight on goals and objectives derived through verbal input) as well as intrinsic or specific factors (e.g., the precise modulation of muscular force achieved through processing kinesthetic input), there is considerable variation in the processes which affect transfer during the various phases of motor learning. According to Gagné and Fleishman (1959), similarity between tasks is the governing factor in positive transfer of learning. Such intertask similarity is based upon three broad considerations: the similarity of the ability constructs common to both tasks, the similarity between the stimulus aspects of the two tasks, and the degree of similarity between the two criterion responses. Each of these three conditions is bounded, however, by the highly specific nature of motor skills themselves.

Buss (1973) has shown that there is a changing pattern in the factor structure of the critical ability constructs required during different phases of skill acquisition. Although all motor skills depend upon extrinsic factors during early learning and upon intrinsic factors in the later phases, two tasks must undergo a series of almost identically corresponding changes in their specific factor structure throughout every phase of the acquisition process if the theory of similar abilities is to provide a viable explanation of transfer of motor learning.

In regard to the role of stimulus similarity in transfer, it has been shown that even in situations in which there are high degrees of similarity between the stimuli (e.g., baseball and softball), differences in the nature of the criterion response result in negative transfer. It is only when nearly identical responses are called for in both situations that stimulus similarity becomes a factor in positive transfer. Response similarity in motor learning is clearly limited by the highly specific nature of motor skills. The specific temporal and spatial patterning of the constituent elements comprising motoric responses virtually precludes any great degree of intertask similarity. Precisely this lack of response similarity accounts for the high degree of negative transfer usually associated with the acquisition of motor skills.

At the initial phase of motor learning, when ideational factors are most important, there is maximum transfer in the learning of such nonspecific factors as the strategies for acquiring the skill. This transfer of knowledge and principles attained in learning prior to the current problem is referred to as nonspecific transfer. It appears ironic, but the activities most facilitated through positive, nonspecific transfer are also the most susceptible to negative transfer between specific elements. In baseball and softball, both activities involve similar strategies and are played with similar implements upon fields that are similarly marked, yet the actual skills in each activity show marked differences in temporal and spatial patterning.

Clearly, the greatest benefits of transfer of learning in the acquisition of motor skills are confined to the earliest levels of learning. This transfer is manifested in the form of learning how to learn and in the resultant development of learning sets. A learning set evolves as a subject becomes familiar with the physical requirements, the procedures followed, and the equipment employed for a particular body of activities. In the baseball-softball analogy, it can be seen that prior knowledge of the principles of softball will clearly facilitate the initial acquisition of baseball skills through the transfer of a number of learning sets. There will be far less uncertainty associated with learning the principles of baseball for an individual with prior softball experience than for an individual with no such experience. The idea of knowing which implements to use and the way in which to use them, as well as knowledge of the overall strategy and purpose of the activity, are practical examples of learning sets which facilitate the initial aspects of motor learning.

Given the highly specific nature of motor skills and the limited effectiveness of nonspecific transfer in the form of learning sets, it seems reasonable to question the applicability of the entire concept of transfer to the learning of motor skills. The true significance of transfer in motor learning is the learner's ability to resist negative transfer between specific skills and maximize the incremental effects of positive transfer. A practical example of this situation is the basketball player who experiences positive, nonspecific transfer of the learning sets associated with a jump shot and a lay-up shot, and simultaneously experiences negative transfer between the patterning of the specific elements of the two skills (e.g., timing and application of muscular force). Although the objectives and strategic considerations are highly similar in both cases, the specific factors in execution are markedly different. The proficient performer is able to resist negative transfer by selecting the appropriate pattern of responses in the exact instant it is called for without any hesitation or spurious activity.

Since the physical educator is teaching complex activities involving substantive levels of nonspecific factors, transfer of learning, even though confined to learning sets, remains a viable area of concern. Such nonspecific transfer in motor learning occurs at different levels. According to Gagné (1970), at least two forms of transfer exist: lateral and vertical. In the lateral transfer of learning, there is a generalization of principles to differing but equally complex learning situations; in vertical transfer of learning, fundamental principles are applied to more highly complex learning situations. Lateral transfer is best exemplified by an actual game situation in which any number of adaptations of basic skills are required. The proficient quarterback is able to adapt his plays to sudden and unexpected changes in the opponent's defensive strategy, as the good hitter in baseball is able to adapt his batting skills to the speed and direction of the various pitches in the pitcher's repertoire. Lateral transfer is a prime requisite in all complex activities since it involves the individual's capacity to relate prior learning to new situations.

The concept of vertical transfer has particular relevance to the role of practice and physical conditioning. One of the basic objectives of physical education is the development of various subroutines requisite to the acquisition of complex activities. Often the acquisition of the subroutines themselves relies upon such physiological factors as the strength and endurance of the muscle groups involved in the execution of the task. The phenomenon of vertical transfer is relevant to all learning situations in which the attainment of the criterion task is contingent upon the prior acquisition of more basic skills. The complex motor activities taught in a physical education program are prime learning situations heavily dependent upon nonspecific vertical transfer of learning. The acquisition of the kip on the horizontal bar, for example, requires sufficient strength in the hip flexor muscles and sufficient flexibility in the hip joint.

When conditions of practice most closely resemble those under which the criterion activity is to be performed, positive, nonspecific lateral transfer is enhanced. This is particularly critical for such factors as the pacing of the activity, the equipment employed in its performance, and the physical characteristics of the practice area. To attain the optimum benefit from a practice session, the activities employed must encompass the widest possible range of conditions likely to be encountered during the actual performance of the criterion skill. Thus, the use of drills or lead-up activities consisting solely of highly stylized, prestructured movements is of questionable value. Although drills which stress dribbling and shooting are essential in developing fundamental basketball skills, a productive practice session must also place these activities in conditions which most closely resemble those prevailing during the actual game situation.

This need to make the practice conditions as identical to the actual criterion conditions (game situation) as possible is primarily related to the lateral aspects of transfer and is therefore most critical when higher levels of proficiency are required. Conversely, when dealing with the low levels of proficiency characteristic of the initial acquisition stages of a task, practice means the development of such nonspecific aspects of proficiency as muscular strength and endurance and patterned sequences of movement subroutines which vertically facilitate the acquisition of the criterion task. Before acquiring a complex task, a student must first acquire a series of relevant basic skills.

### Measuring Transfer

In order to understand the role of transfer in motor learning, objective indices must be developed which can assess its degree and its direction. Ellis (1965) provides a number of formulas which can be applied to the acquisition of complex motor skills. The first formula is applicable to situations in which proficiency in the performance of the transfer task is indicated by an increasing score, such as the amount of distance covered in a throw or a jump, or the number of points scored. It is expressed symbolically as $\frac{E-C}{C} \times 100$, with E representing the mean score of the experimental group and C representing the mean score of the control group.

A second form of design for measuring transfer is used when superior performance is indicated by a decreasing score, as in the use of the time or number of trials to reach a given criterion of learning, or by the number of erroneous responses elicited during the practice session. this transfer design is symbolically represented by the formula $\frac{C-E}{C} \times 100$.

If a physical educator were interested in the effects of bilateral transfer upon the acquisition of an eye-hand coordination task, either formula might be used. If the interest were in the total score achieved by the experimental group, the first formula would be used. In this hypothetical example, the experimental group has had prior practice on the criterion eye-hand coordination task with the nonfavored hand, and the control group has had none. Comparing the performance of both groups on the criterion measure (performance on the eye-hand coordination task with the favored hand), one finds that the experimental group has scored an average of 50 points, the mean score of the control group is 30 points. Substitute the data in the formula $\frac{E-C}{C} \times 100$ and the percentage of positive transfer is equal to $\frac{50-30}{30} \times 100$ or 66 percent. Suppose that the researcher were not concerned with the actual scores achieved by the subjects, but rather with the time or number of trials it took the subjects to reach some predetermined criterion of learning. Hypothesize that the experimental group acquired the task in an average of 75 trials as compared to a mean of 100 trials for the control group and substitute these values in the formula $\frac{C-E}{C} \times 100$. The percentage of positive transfer is equal to $\frac{100-75}{75} \times 100$ or 33 percent.

Since the first transfer formula is employed in situations where superior performance is indicated by an increasing score, if the mean score of the control group had been greater than the mean score of the experimental group, negative transfer would have resulted. Since the second transfer formula is employed in situations where superior performance is indicated by a decreasing score, if the mean score of the experimental group had been greater than that of the control group, negative transfer would have resulted. (See Chapter 3 for a discussion of the appropriate statistical techniques employed in assessing the significance of these observed differences.)

### Intersegmental Transfer

A problem often associated with the broad theoretical issues of motor learning concerns the transfer of skilled performance between two different segments of the body. This transfer may involve contralateral segments in the same hemisphere (right and left arm or right and left leg), ipsilateral segments in different body hemispheres (right leg and right arm or left leg and left arm), or contralateral segments in different hemispheres (left leg and right arm or right leg and left arm). This intersegmental transfer is variously referred to as bilateral transfer, cross-member transfer, or cross-education. Ammons (1958), after intensively reviewing the literature, developed a taxonomy governing the critical factors in bilateral transfer. The elements that tended to result in the highest levels of cross-member transfer were nonspecific in nature: warm-up decrement, temporary work decrement, or proficiency. In addition, motivational and emotional factors, prior experience, and methodological and strategic considerations all tended to transfer in a bilateral fashion.

Ammons also observed that there tends to be a greater degree of positive transfer when one task is performed by two different body segments than when two different though highly similar tasks are executed with the same body segment. Such bilateral transfer is considered incomplete, however, because the degree of skill transferred is always less than the original level of proficiency. Differences in the factor structure of specific skills also affect the level of cross-member transfer attained. Skills that are low in complexity are apt to yield higher levels of bilateral transfer than highly complex tasks. Cross-transfer is also a directional phenomenon in that there is always greater transfer between the favored and the nonfavored limb than there is between the nonfavored and the favored limb segments.

Dunham (1977b) studied the effects of bilateral transfer on the performance of a pursuit-rotor tracking task but failed to confirm the findings of Ammons. Dunham observed no significant differences in transfer, no matter which hand (preferred or nonpreferred) was employed initially. Kohl and Roenker (1980), in contrast, observed significant positive transfer from right- to left-hand rotary pursuit skill under conditions of mental rehearsal and physical practice. To obviate depression resulting from the accumulation of work decrement (a factor absent in mental practice), the authors conducted a second experiment in which interpolated rest periods dissipated the decremental factor. As in the former study, significant bilateral transfer was observed under mental as well as physical practice conditions. The authors conclude that, in the case of rotary pursuit tracking, mental practice can facilitate bilateral transfer of skill.

There is greater cross-member transfer between contralateral segments in the same hemisphere (right and left hand) than between ipsilateral segments in different hemispheres (right hand and right foot). This phenomenon is attributable to the similarity in the basic movement patterns and to the degree of morphological homology associated with corresponding limb segments that are bilaterally symmetrical. The right and left hand, for example, are anatomically structured to execute identical functions; the hand and foot are clearly structured for different functions. In summarizing the phenomenon of bilateral transfer, one sees that although evidence exists in its support, it is largely confined to the nonspecific aspects of motor skill acquisition and in many situations may be a mere artifactual effect of variations and weakness in experimental design.

Dunham (1977a) writes that many skills which are performed on both sides of the body involve a component called coincidence/anticipation (C/A). It is defined as the ability to intercept accurately a moving object at a designated point. This ability is believed fundamental to the successful performance of such diverse skills as soccer (dribbling, trapping, and kicking), handball (returning a serve), and basketball (dribbling and shooting). The author studied performance upon a simple C/A task with the right foot, supplemented by practice with the left foot. The latter did not facilitate the former. Dunham writes that these findings apparently contrast with the majority of studies on bilateral transfer phenomena, but accord with those of prior studies of coincidence/anticipation which have indicated that significant improvements have been confined to the early stages of practice. Dunham argues that subjects were able to monitor and regulate performance in order to achieve maximal levels of proficiency that could not significantly be affected by subsequent practice.

*Implications for Teaching*

The role of transfer constitutes a critical factor in all forms of learning; prior experience can facilitate or inhibit the acquisition of a given task. The study of transfer in the area of motor learning is complicated by the highly specific nature of motor skills themselves. The initial phase of skill acquisition is dependent upon such nonspecific factors as understanding the rules and principles which govern the performance of the task. The later phase, devoted to the attainment of advanced levels of proficiency, depends upon the learner's capacity to integrate precisely temporal and spatial information in the execution of specific response patterns.

Since the initial phase of skill acquisition embodies general nonspecific factors, the early learning of a motor skill may well appear to be facilitated by the prior acquisition of an overtly similar activity (positive transfer). During the later phases of the acquisition, however, it is most probable that the individual with prior experience may manifest errors which will ultimately depress performance to a level well below that of the individual with no prior experience (negative transfer). Positive and negative transfer are, therefore, relative rather than absolute concepts since every motor learning situation possesses the potential for the occurrence of either of these two alternative outcomes. If a given learning situation will yield positive or negative transfer depends upon the perceived environmental consequences of the response. If performance upon the transfer task is facilitated despite the negative interference effects resulting from the initial task, then the net result is positive transfer. If interference outweighs facilitation, negative transfer results.

The greater the similarity between the initial task and the transfer task, the greater the likelihood of negative transfer. Such negative transfer usually manifests itself in the form of a hybrid response bearing properties of the initial and the transfer tasks. The greater the similarity between the hybrid response and the desired response, the greater the difficulty in detecting the error and effecting the appropriate adjustments in the response pattern. While it has become almost axiomatic that one should "teach for transfer," current evidence dealing with the nature of skill acquisition pragmatically indicates that a teacher of motor skills should actually strive to minimize negative transfer rather than attempt to maximize positive transfer.

A major application of the principles of transfer is to lead-up activities. The stated purpose of a lead-up is to provide the learner with an activity overtly similar to the criterion task but much less complex in nature. Prime examples of such activities are the dribble and lay-up drills used in teaching fundamental basketball skills and practicing the criterion skill at rates of speed considerably lower than those employed in the actual game situation (practicing at "three-quarter speed"). While these less complex preparatory activities may at first appear to facilitate the acquisition of the criterion task, in the end, the greater the differences in temporal patterning between the practice task and the criterion, the greater the degree of interference and negative transfer the learner will experience.

Another application of transfer principles is to the nature of the criterion activity. If the criterion skill is a Level III activity, practice sessions which stress Level I activities have little relevance to the actual learning situation. In order for practice to facilitate the acquisition of the criterion task, its conditions must closely resemble those of the criterion situation.

### References

Ammons, R.B. "Le Mouvement." *In* G.S. and J.P. Seward (eds.), *Current Psychological Issues.* New York: Henry Holt, 1958.

———, C.H.Ammons, and R. L. Morgan. "Transfer of Skill and Decremental Factors Along the Speed Dimension in Rotary Pursuit." *Perceptual and Motor Skills, 6* (1956), 43.

Baker, K.E., R.C. Wylie, and R.M. Gagné. "Transfer of Training to a Motor Skill As a Function of Variation in Rate of Response." *Journal of Experimental Psychology, 40* (1950), 721– 732.

Boswell, J.J. and A.L. Irion. "Transfer of Training As a Function of Target Speed in Pursuit-Rotor Performance: Proactive and Retroactive Effects." *Journal of Motor Behavior, 7* (1975), 105–111.

Buss, A.R. "Learning Transfer and Ability Factors: A Multivariate Model." *Psychological Bulletin, 80* (1973), 106–112.

Cratty, B.J. *Movement Behavior and Motor Learning.* 3rd ed. Philadelphia: Lea and Febiger, 1973.

Davies, D.R. "The Effects of Tuition Upon the Process of Learning a Complex Motor Skill." *In* R.N. Singer (ed.), *Readings in Motor Learning.* Philadelphia: Lea and Febiger, 1972.

Day, R.H. "Relative Task Difficulty and Transfer of Training in Skilled Performance." *Psychological Bulletin, 53* (1956), 160–168.

Deese, J. *The Psychology of Learning.* 2nd ed. New York: McKay, 1958.

Dey, M.K. "Influence of Response Similarity on Interferences in Perceptual Motor Learning." *Journal of Motor Behavior, 9* (1977), 95– 100.

Dickinson, J. and N. Higgins. "Release from Proactive and Retroactive Interference in Motor Short-Term Memory." *Journal of Motor Behavior, 9* (1977), 61–66.

Dunham, P. "Effect of Bilateral Transfer on Coincidence/Anticipation Performance." *Research Quarterly, 48* (1977a), 51– 55.

————. "Effect of Practice Order on the Efficiency of Bilateral Skill Acquisition." *Research Quarterly, 48* (1977b), 284–287.

Ellis, H.C. *The Transfer of Learning.* New York: Macmillan, 1965.

Fitts, P.M. "Perceptual-Motor Skill Learning." *In* A.W. Melton (ed.), *Categories of Human Learning,* New York: Academic Press, 1964.

Fleishman, E.A. "Individual Differences and Motor Learning." *In* R.M. Gagné (ed.), *Learning and Individual Differences.* Columbus, Ohio: Merrill, 1967.

———— and S. Rich. "The Role of Kinesthetic and Spatial-Visual Ability in Perceptual-Motor Learning." *Journal of Experimental Psychology,* 56 (1963), 6–11.

Gagné, R.M. *The Conditions of Learning.* 2nd ed. New York: Holt, Rinehart and Winston, 1970.

————, K.E. Baker, and H. Foster. "On the Relation Between Similarity and Transfer of Training in the Learning of Discriminative Motor Tasks." *Psychological Review, 57* (1950), 67–79.

———— and E.A. Fleishman. *Psychology and Human Performance.* New York: Henry Holt, 1959.

Granit, R. *The Basis of Motor Control*. New York: Academic Press, 1970.

Henry, F.M. "Specificity vs. Generality in Learning Motor Skills." *Proceedings of the College Physical Education Association, 61* (1958), 126–128.

Hicks, R.E. and D.M. Cohn. "Lack of Proactive Inhibition in a Psychomotor Task at Two Retention Intervals." *Journal of Motor Behavior, 7* (1975), 101–104.

Hinrichs, J.R. "Ability Correlates in Learning a Psychomotor Task." *Journal of Applied Psychology, 54* (1970), 56–64.

Holding, D.H. "Transfer Between Difficult and Easy Tasks." *British Journal of Psychology, 53* (1962), 397–407.

———. "An Approximate Transfer Surface." *Journal of Motor Behavior, 8* (1976), 1–9.

Irion, A.L. "A Brief History of Research on the Acquisition of Skill." *In* E.A. Bilodeau (ed.), *Acquisition of Skill*. New York: Academic Press, 1966.

Jensen, B.E. "Pretask Speed Training and Movement Complexity." *Research Quarterly, 47* (1976), 657–665.

Kohl, R.M. and D.L. Roenker. "Bilateral Transfer As a Function of Mental Imagery." *Journal of Motor Behavior, 12* (1980), 197–206.

Livesey, J.P. and J.I. Laszlo. "Effect of Task Similarity on Transfer Performance." *Journal of Motor Behavior, 11* (1979), 11–21.

McGeoch, J.A. and A.L. Irion. *The Psychology of Human Learning*. 2nd ed. New York: McKay, 1961.

Mohr, D.R. and M.E. Barrett. "Effects of Knowledge of Mechanical Principles in Learning to Perform Intermediate Swimming Skills." *In* R.N. Singer (ed.), *Readings in Motor Learning*. Philadelphia: Lea and Febiger, 1972.

Nelson, D.O. "Studies of Transfer of Learning in Gross Motor Skills." *Research Quarterly, 28* (1957), 364–373.

Osgood, C.E. "The Similarity Paradox in Human Learning: A Resolution." *Psychological Review, 56* (1949), 132–143.

Rivenes, R.S. and C.S. Caplan. "Concurrent Task Practice Conditions and Transfer." *Perceptual and Motor Skills, 34* (1972), 941–942.

Sage, G.H. and J.E. Hornak. "Progressive Speed Practice in Learning a Continuous Motor Skill." *Research Quarterly, 49* (1978), 190–196.

# CHAPTER 5

# Distribution of Practice

THE PROBLEM OF ESTABLISHING the length and distribution of the practice period, in terms of the initial scheduling of activities throughout the semester and the temporal distribution of work and rest within each respective class session, is often subordinated to considerations which are more practical than theoretical in their nature. Controversy exists over the actual effects of distribution of practice on learning. Theorists have held that learning works best in distributed rather than massed practice, given an identical total amount of practice time, but empirical evidence does not consistently substantiate this superiority. This lack of consistency may be attributed to three factors.

First, there is the problem of definition. Neither massed nor distributed practice can be defined in absolute terms since both are relative to the length and frequency of work and rest periods in any given learning situation. Massed practice requires continual response for a set amount of time, a set number of trials, or until some predetermined criterion of learning is reached within a *single* practice session. Distributed practice involves a *series* of practice sessions consisting of a set number of trials or some set amount of time separated by rest periods of a predetermined interval. Empirical investigations into the effects of distribution of practice upon motor learning have yielded diverse findings because the temporal distribution of the work and rest periods differed. For instance, experiments using a design in which short work periods are followed by brief rest periods have yielded far different results from studies in which long work periods are separated by long periods of rest.

Secondly, there are questions regarding the nature of the experimental learning task itself—is it verbal or motor, and if a motor task, does it involve fine motor or gross motor abilities? Is it continuous or discrete in nature? Studies on distributed practice using motor tasks have differed in results from studies using verbal tasks, as have experiments conducted on fine motor tasks from those using gross motor tasks, or discrete tasks from continuous tasks.

Lastly, there are the variations in theoretical approach. Theoretical explanations of the superiority of distributed over massed practice sessions may be divided into three groups: 1) those dealing with

111

inhibition and performance decrement; 2) those hypothesizing preservation, consolidation, and maturation; and 3) those favoring differential forgetting. Each theory, however, has a limited application, and no one theory can account for the effect of distribution of practice on the acquisition and performance of diverse learning tasks. This need not be a major problem, if one can link the various theories with definite types of learning tasks. In motor learning, inhibition theory has provided the most plausible explanation for the superiority of distributed over massed practice. Differential forgetting theories only have application in verbal learning; consolidation theories in both.

### Theoretical Issues

Research on the effects of distribution of practice on skill learning has undergone considerable transition from its inception at the beginning of the century to the present. Irion (1966) has identified three distinct periods in the history of skill acquisition research which reflect changing theoretical approaches to experimentation in this area.

The early period during the first three decades of this century was primarily concerned with postulating a universal rule governing the effects of distribution of practice. Once this rule had been formulated, it would then have been theoretically possible to design optimum work and rest schedules for an infinite variety of tasks. The research of this period primarily manipulated the three basic variables in distribution of practice experimentation: amount of practice, length of rest, and total time elapsed.

The middle period ranged from the 1930s to the 1950s and was characterized by changes in the theoretical approach to the problem. The factor of fatigue was superseded by such intervening constructs as maturation, rehearsal, and neural consolidation.

The third period of research, from the 1950s to the present, has introduced new theoretical formulations of reactive inhibition, conditioned inhibition, and reminiscence, and their specific application to motor learning. These theoretical advances were accomplished by a major change in thinking about practice distribution, i.e., that it affects performance only. The decremental effects of massing of practice are temporary, rather than permanent as was previously believed.

Irion (1953) writes that Hull's two-factor inhibition theory has provided one of the more satisfactory explanations to date of the reminiscence phenomenon,* which is often concomitant with distributed

---

*An increase in the proficiency of a partially learned act which is attributable to the effects of an interpolated rest period.

practice in human motor learning. According to Hull (1952), there are two types of inhibition, reactive $^{I}R$ and conditioned $s^{I}R$. It is Hull's position that every response carries with it some degree of inhibitory potential which accumulates with each response. This leads to a decrement in performance and the eventual total cessation of the response. Hull described this phenomenon of reactive inhibition as a negative, fatigue-like drive which accumulates with work and dissipates with rest. The phenomenon of reminiscence has often been interpreted as the result of reactive inhibition dissipation which occurs during the rest period interpolated into a distributed practice session. This results in an increment in performance on the trial following rest. (For elaboration, see Specificity of Reminiscence later in this chapter.) A familiar example of this phenomenon is the basketball player who finds that after a long practice session he is missing an ever-increasing number of shots. If the player takes a rest and then resumes practice, his performance is often improved.

The second factor in Hull's inhibition theory is conditioned inhibition which he describes as habit. If reactive inhibition is allowed to accumulate, as is the case in massed practice, it builds to the point where the subject eventually ceases to respond. It is this cessation of response in the presence of the stimulus of the learning situation which leads to conditioned inhibition. According to Hull, any response which reduces a drive is defined as a reinforcer. Therefore, stoppage in work (a reinforcer) caused by accumulated reactive inhibition (the drive) will strengthen the tendency of a subject's resting response to become conditioned to the practice task itself (the stimulus).

An example of this phenomenon may be seen in the over-zealous coach who forces his players to practice without rest intervals. Inevitably, a player will stop for a rest, but upon so doing will be immediately derided by the coach and urged in no uncertain terms to resume practice. If this process is repeated often enough, the player in question should theoretically develop a lack of concentration and ultimately manifest a lazy "turned-off" attitude whenever confronted by the practice situation.

Consolidation theory concerns itself with hypothetical learning variables. The classical preservation theory set forth by Muller and Pilzecker (Dore and Hilgard, 1938) assumes that the neural activity involved in learning persists for some time after the cessation of formal practice. Massing of practice does not give time for the preservative "setting in" of the neural traces which takes place during the rest period. This premise accounts for the phenomenon of reminiscence and the superiority of distribution of practice.

The rehearsal theory, as discussed by Richardson (1972), is a type of preservation theory which identifies the preservative process as implicit practice or rehearsal during the rest period. This theory holds that gains which have been attributed to practice actually occurred during the rest period in an unmeasured and uncontrolled fashion. Viewed thusly, rehearsal is a possible correlate of reminiscence. Objections to this theory are based upon results of experiments favoring distribution over massing of practice using animals and of studies of human motor learning on the pursuit rotor. In the first case, active rehearsal cannot be reasonably assumed, and in the second, implicit practice is ineffective due to a lack of symbolic attributes of the task.

Current theoretical approaches to the problem of learning look upon rehearsal as a factor in the memory of verbal and sensory information. Rehearsal may be defined as the repeated passage of a bit of information through the same limited capacity channel (Coombs et al., 1970). If this channel is interfered with by the presence of new information, preventing rehearsal, forgetting of the original information will occur.

Current interpretations of rehearsal theory applied to distribution of practice and skill learning produce a quite different set of predictions about the effects of massed practice on learning. Kintsch (1970), for example, distinguished a short-term memory store and a sensory memory store. The sensory data could be stored for a very brief period without being analyzed (rehearsed). Unlike verbal information, which is forgotten due to interference, sensory data decays quickly with time alone. Since the storage of sensory information is relatively free from the effects of interference, massed practice on a redundant motor task should sustain the sensory input over time and facilitate its retention. Conversely, a distributed practice period should inhibit the process by increasing the decay of sensory memory during the rest periods. In motor learning, the sensory data is comprised of proprioceptive feedback information.

The stimulus maturation theory of Wheeler and Perkins (Dore and Hilgard, 1937) asserts that the rate of improvement in a learned task should be a function of the time elapsed from the beginning of practice rather than the number of trials occurring within that time. It is reasoned by Wheeler that the "preservating process" is a form of growth maturation induced by stimulation but relatively independent of rate of stimulation. This hypothesis can apply only within the limits of comparatively short-increment rest periods. If the trials are spaced at very large intervals, the rate of improvement will be greatly impeded or even halted due to the effects of interference and forgetting.

The theory of differential forgetting, as proposed by McGeoch and Irion (1961), deals only with the effects of distribution of practice on verbal learning. It is predicated upon two positions: errors are less well learned than correct responses, which are repeatedly reinforced; and a lapse of time will permit the errors to be forgotten more rapidly than the correct responses. Hence, distributed practice will be more advantageous than massed practice.

### The Learning-Performance Distinction

Thus far, the discussion has been largely confined to theories on the superiority of distributed practice. There are, however, several additional factors influencing the outcome of research on the effects of massing of practice. Researchers and theorists, for example, have often separated learning and performance when discussing the effects of distributed practice. Learning is regarded as actual habit strength measured in terms of the resistance of a given response to extinction or the latency or time interval between the presentation of the stimulus and the emission of the response. Performance, on the other hand, is evaluated in terms of an organism's characteristic emitted responses, for example the frequency and the amplitude of responding at a given temporal point. According to this behavioristic position, learning sets the theoretical upper limit of performance. In motor learning, however, performance and learning are interrelated to such a high degree that performance becomes the criterion for learning.

Inhibition theories, or theories of performance decrement, postulate that massing of practice affects only the variables of performance but not the habit strength or learning variables. The interpolated rest periods in a distributed practice session allow for the dissipation of accumulated inhibitory potential which temporarily depresses performance. The longer the practice period and the greater the effort required to perform the task, the higher the level of accumulated inhibition. According to inhibition theorists, it is this inhibition dissipation during rest which accounts for the phenomenon of reminiscence and for the superiority of distribution over massing of practice.

Maturation theorists, on the other hand, hold that the temporal distribution of work and rest periods affects the actual learning or habit strength developed as a result of practice, i.e., that the degree of learning is a function of the total time (including rest) the subject spends at a given learning task until a predetermined criterion of performance is attained. These theories stress that stimulus traces persist after practice ceases. During rest, these traces are "preserved" or "consolidated," resulting in the continuation of learning after the cessation of practice. Since the actual total practice time is usually identical for distributed and massed practice groups during an experiment, the subjects learning under conditions of distributed practice have, according to maturation theorists, a greater total time in which to learn because the rest periods and the practice periods are equally important.

As stated before, performance and learning are so highly interrelated in motor learning that one cannot rule out inhibition theories from partially accounting for the superiority of distributed over massed practice. By the same token, maturation theories may also partially account for the phenomenon of reminiscence, often concomitant with distributed practice for motor skill acquisition.

### Experimental Findings

Experimental research on the effects of practice distribution upon the acquisition of motor skills has yielded conflicting results. Differences in such factors as the nature of the criterion task, the temporal patterning of the work and rest periods, and the criteria of learning employed in a given study complicate rather than simplify the issue. Dore and Hilgard (1937), employing a pursuit-rotor tracking task, observed that a rest period of eleven minutes resulted in better performance than three minutes or one minute, the latter being the least effective. Predicated upon these findings, the authors proposed that learning is more closely related to the total time elapsed from the beginning of practice (including rest periods) than to the actual amount of practice itself.

This position was substantiated by the findings of Duncan (1951), who observed that by keeping the total length of the practice period (rest period and actual practice time) constant, subjects working under distributed practice conditions performed significantly better upon a pursuit-rotor task than subjects who had received 66 percent more actual practice under massed conditions. A further substantiation of the conclusions of Dore and Hilgard was offered by Harmon and Miller (1950), who observed that in pursuit-rotor tracking performance, the length of the time between practice periods can prove just as important as the length of the actual practice period itself.

Travis (1936) provided evidence which cast doubt upon the assumption that learning is a function of total time rather than of actual practice trials. He found that a rest period of twenty minutes resulted in significantly better performance upon a pursuit-rotor task than rest periods of five minutes, forty-eight hours, seventy-two hours, or 120 hours. In addition to the observation that the longest rest did not produce the best results, Travis found that the insertion of a one-minute rest period between two-minute work periods resulted in a constant rise in performance.* These findings led to the conclusion that, at least in the case of pursuit-rotor tracking, it is short-term rest periods that facilitate performance.

Further evidence supporting the superiority of short rest periods was given by Cook and Hilgard (1949), who found that by progressively increasing rest periods for one experimental group (twenty seconds, one minute, three minutes) and decreasing them for the other group (three minutes, one minute, twenty seconds), the group with decreasing rest periods significantly outperformed the other group on a pursuit-rotor task. These differences were confined to the first day of practice only; no significant differences existed between groups at the end of the study. Cook and Hilgard's principal observation is that following long rests, performance tends to be alike, regardless of the arrangement of prior practice.

The preceding studies all involved pursuit-rotor tracking tasks, but investigations into the effects of practice distribution use such diverse activities as: 1) fine coordinated movements, such as pattern tracing and mirror drawing; 2) finger maze tracing; 3) gross motor response to a stimulus, such as pushing a button or stepping on a pedal in response to a buzzer, light, or electric shock; 4) eye-hand coordination, such as throwing an object at a target; and 5) specific sport skills. Studies employing one type of task and those employing differing tasks yield conflicting results. Cook (1944), for example, found massed practice superior to distributed practice for two types of maze learning. Franklin and Brozek (1947) found no differences between massed and distributed practice in the learning of a gross motor task (response to a light stimulus while walking on a treadmill) and a fine motor task (pattern tracing). It was also observed that the spacing of practice (regular or irregular) had no effect upon the performance of either task.

Harmon and Crendine (1961), studying the effects of practice distribution upon the learning of a mirror tracing task, observed significant differences in favor of the massed practice group during the initial phases of the study; as proficiency developed, however, all groups progressed at the same rate. The phenomenon of reminiscence was not observed. Proficiency which developed late in the practice period did not carry over to the succeeding practice session. There were also no long-term effects of the temporal distribution of the practice sessions; no significant differences in performance existed between the massed and distributed practice groups on a retention test given three weeks after the final practice.

---

*Groups having continuous practice periods for the same total length of time manifested a consistent decrease in performance.

Knapp and Dixon (1950) studied the effects of practice period duration on learning to juggle. Subjects practicing for five minutes and resting for 24 hours performed significantly better than subjects who practiced for 15 minutes and rested for 48 hours. Analyzing these findings in light of the conclusions shed by related research, the authors contend that there are seven factors which influence the effects of practice distribution: 1) duration of the practice period; 2) length of rest; 3) practice method; 4) speed of movement; 5) characteristics of the learner (individual differences); 6) activity of the learner between practice periods (interpolated activities); and 7) complexity of the skill (task taxonomy).

Singer (1965) studied the effects of practice distribution upon the performance of a novel basketball skill* and found distributed practice superior. On a retention test given a month after the cessation of the experiment, however, the performance of the massed practice group was significantly better than it was at the conclusion of the study; that of the distributed practice group declined. Singer attributed these findings to the accumulation of reactive inhibition, which depressed performance. This decrement is only temporary since reactive inhibition dissipates if a rest period of sufficient duration is provided.

Additional research using gross motor skills has yielded conflicting results. Young (1954) found that a four-day-per-week distribution of practice facilitated the learning of archery. Badminton responded to a two-day-per-week distribution. Knapp (1966) cites studies by Cozens and Scott that ranked distributed practice superior to massed in the learning of track and swimming skills. Caron (1970) also obtained significant differences favoring distributed practice for the performance of a peg-turning task by college males, and Austin (1975) found the same for the acquisition of a task requiring throwing for velocity. Stelmach (1968) found no significant differences in the rates of learning for massed and distributed practice groups performing two gross motor tasks (a stabilimeter balance task and a free-standing ladder climb); Kleinman (1976), the same for basic gymnastic skills.

A final example of dissension among practice distribution studies is found in Mohr's intensive review of research in this area. Mohr (1960) reports the following studies on distribution of practice using physical education skills.

1. Niemeyer found that in the early learning of swimming, badminton, and volleyball skills, distributed practice sessions of 30 minutes, three times per week, were better than massed practice for 60 minutes, twice a week.

---

*The subjects had to get the ball through the basket by bouncing it off the floor.

2. Miller, using four groups of college women, had nine practice periods of 50 shots each in learning the fundamentals of billiards. One group had practice one day per week, a second three days per week, a third had daily practice, and the fourth had progressively longer time intervals between practice days. The only significant differences, however, were in favor of the fourth group.
3. Lashley found that several distributed practice sessions yielded more effective results than fewer periods of greater duration in the learning of archery and rifle shooting.
4. Webster investigated the length and interval of the practice period in learning bowling and reported that shorter and more frequent practice sessions are more effective.

*Specificity of Reminiscence*

Several factors are common to the relationship between performance level on a given task and the temporal distribution of practice. Tasks which are well learned, simple in nature, externally paced, and temporally distributed in a manner in which work periods of one to two minutes are separated by rest periods of thirty seconds to one minute appear most prone to the adverse effects of massing of practice. Conversely, the acquisition of new, highly complex tasks which are subject paced and temporally distributed in a manner in which practice periods of thirty minutes to one hour are separated by rest periods of twenty-four to forty-eight hours appears to be minimally affected by massing of practice (Purohit, 1968). These observations are reducible to three main conditions.

The first is concerned with the continuous or discrete nature of the task. Continuous tasks generally tend to be more coherent (Fitts, 1964) and, hence, appear more susceptible to the effects of massed practice. Noble et al. (1979) write that work periods interspersed with intervals of rest (distributed practice) will, in most cases, produce higher levels of performance on tasks requiring continual response than extended practice periods without rest (massed practice). This relationship between temporal distribution of practice and level of proficiency does not hold in the case of tasks requiring discrete responses.

The second involves the differences which characterize fine motor tasks and gross motor tasks. Most experimentation on distribution of practice has used fine motor tasks of low complexity. Gross motor tasks are comprised of movement patterns involving large segments of the body (e.g., limb and trunk movements in which strength, endurance, and flexibility are important). Fine motor tasks are usually confined to movements of the arms, wrists, hands, and fingers and are usually dependent upon eye-hand coordination and limb steadiness (Fleishman, 1967).

The third and last condition is the issue of the learning-performance distinction. According to Eysenck (1964), consolidation theories and inhibition theories may account for the phenomenon of reminiscence. Consolidation theories have been employed to study the effects of practice distribution on learning variables; inhibition theories, on performance variables.

Eysenck (1965) feels that "this is an important distinction in all modern learning theories, and the failure in much recent thinking to preserve the difference between performance and learning in reminiscence may be responsible for the apparent failure of prediction." He cautions that reminiscence is specific and varies in degree according to the nature and complexity of the criterion task, the motivational and ability levels of the subjects, and whether the study involves learning or performance variables. Eysenck's contention is substantiated, at least in part, by inconsistency in the findings of studies based on criterion measures other than pursuit-rotor tracking.

Ammons (1947) agrees that the effects of practice distribution are most pronounced during the initial stages of learning a new motor skill, when blocks of trials are separated by rest periods of several minutes duration. The increment in performance from prerest to postrest practice (reminiscence) has been attributed to many diverse theoretical factors: maturation, differential forgetting, memory trace consolidation, the dissipation of reactive inhibition ($I_R$). Ammons contends that theories which stress either consolidation or the dissipation of $I_R$ are the most realistic explanations of reminiscence.

There is still controversy over the degree to which $I_R$ and reminiscence itself are task specific. Huang and Payne (1977) write that there is empirical evidence to support the contention that both factors are specific in nature since reminiscence has been observed even when the rest interval is filled with a competing activity. These findings imply that $I_R$ is specific to the principal task but independent of the interpolated activity. The authors argue, however, that no definitive statement can be made about the specificity of $I_R$. There is considerable counter-evidence indicating that reminiscence is partially or wholly blocked when alternative activities are interpolated into the rest interval.

Hsu and Payne (1979), for example, observed no reminiscence upon a criterion task (right-handed mirror tracing) following a period filled with an interpolated activity (right-handed pursuit-rotor tracking). Reminiscence upon the criterion task was observed, however, when the interpolated activity was left-handed pursuit-rotor tracking. The authors contend that reminiscence may be specific to the involved limb segment rather than to the learning task. Catalano (1978) observed reminiscence for the continuous task of pursuit-rotor tracking following an inter-polated rest period, but an interpolated rest period for a discrete task (lever positioning) resulted in performance decrement. Ammons (1947) argues that reminiscence is a complex phenomenon which may involve several factors, each of which may vary in terms of the nature of the criterion task and the stage of the learning process.

The lack of consistent findings from studies of practice distribution effects upon the learning and performance of sport skills may well have to do with differences in the taxonomy of the particular activities employed. Skills which are discrete and intrinsically paced may be inherently distributed, thereby precluding the detrimental effects of massed practice.

It is evident from the preceding discussion that experimental results obtained from studies on learned, uncomplex, continuous, fine motor tasks serve as poor predictors for the outcome of experimentation on gross motor skill acquisition. Skill acquisition has been divided into three stages by Fitts (1962). (See Chapter 2, p.52.) Experimentation on distribution of practice employing simple tasks which have been already acquired by the subject deals with the third stage of skill acquisition, the slow steady increase in performance characteristic of the stage of automation of execution. In contrast, when studying the effects of distribution on the acquisition of complex gross motor tasks such as gymnastic skills, one is dealing with the second stage of skill acquisition in which the subject is learning to identify and discriminate proprio-ceptive cues and, as a result, to adjust and modify his responses by appropriate changes in the magnitude and direction of the forces he is exerting.

### Locus of Control

The neuroanatomical processes central to the performance of a familiar, well-learned task differ from those underlying the trial-and-error approach which characterizes the acquisition period for a new and unfamiliar skill. In the former, the subject is processing familiar or redundant information through already established channels (Attneave, 1959). In the latter, the subject is processing unfamiliar and unpredictable information, in which case, the subject must discern the relevant cues from this information in order to establish the appropriate neurological channels for successful execution of the task. Hence, it may be concluded that research on the effects of distribution of practice on the performance of an already learned task will not predict the outcome on unlearned tasks. This conclusion is supported, in part, by Fleishman (1960), who found that abilities contributing to performance during the initial stages of skill acquisition differ from those critical to later learning.

A possible explanation for the apparent lack of agreement between findings of gross motor task and fine motor task studies may lie in the fact that fine movement patterns have a different neuroanatomical locus than gross motor patterns. Evidence for this position is given by Smith (1966). (See Chapter 2, p.48 for his analysis of motion and Chapter 6 for a detailed discussion of the neurophysiological aspects of motor learning.) Smith and Smith (1966) write that "experimental analyses have revealed that the different movement components have specialized properties and are independently variable in performance and learning." Their specialization and relative independence are attributable to their differential regulation by distinctive neural mechanisms. Patterned motion, however, is never completely independent. It is characterized by the precise integration of the various components with reference to each other and to the overall pattern. It is assumed, therefore, that specialized centers exist in the brain for the purpose of integrating postural and transport movements and transport and manipulative movements.

A major aspect of skill acquisition is improvement in the precision and efficiency of these integrations. Relating the preceding discussion to the problems of experimentation on the effects of distribution of practice, one can hypothesize that different motor tasks vary in their susceptibility to massing of practice just as they vary in their neuroanatomical complexity and organization. A final argument in substantiation of this position is based upon the factor analytic work of Fleishman on the differentiation of basic motor abilities.

### Individual Differences

According to Fleishman (1964), factors represent clusters or groupings of tests. First, a number of tests are given. A proportion of these tests may be observed to correlate highly with one another but have very low or zero correlation with the remaining tests. Another grouping of tests may correlate highly with one another and have poor correlation with the first cluster. In this case, two distinct clusters have been identified. Fleishman argues that an average score on the first grouping of tests and the same on the second grouping would represent an individual's score on two separate factors having very low correlation with one another. Using this approach, Fleishman postulates the existence of two distinguishable areas of motor ability: fine manipulative ability and gross motor ability. To support his position, he argues that these areas have been separated in order to indicate that they are distinct from one another in terms of correlations between measures of individual differences. In essence, there is little correlation between a subject's performance in the two areas; hence, each area supports a different kind of motor performance (Gagné and Fleishman, 1959).

Noble (1978) writes that, while practice in and of itself is essential to the acquisition of motor skills, pretask ability factors, through their interaction with the conditions of practice and the nature of the learning task, are critical determinants of rates of gain and final levels of proficiency. Fleishman (1966) discusses findings which indicate that if the experimenter knows the subjects' previously developed abilities, accurate prediction of later performance under massed and distributed practice is enhanced. Fleishman's position concerning the relationship between pretask individual difference and the effects of distribution of practice is substantiated by the findings of Boswell and Spatz (1975). They observed poor correlation between prerest and postrest performance on a standard U.S. Air Force 60 rpm pursuit rotor by right-handed college males. They contend that this poor relationship is independent of the amount of prerest practice and results instead from variability in the levels of particular organismic factors or abilities which affect an individual's capacity to dissipate reactive inhibition ($I_R$).

Further evidence supporting the position that reminiscence is influenced by pretask individual differences is provided by Payne and Huang (1977), who observed differences in reminiscence related to the subjects' sex and the particular criterion tasks. McBride and Payne (1979) cite evidence for a significant interaction between age, sex, and task-related variables and the amount of reminiscence. Young adult females demonstrated greater levels of reminiscence than male subjects in the same age group while performing rotary pursuit and mirror-tracing tasks. Prepubescent females performing these same tasks, however, demonstrated less reminiscence than their male counterparts. The authors report that, when the criterion task involved reversed alphabet printing, there were no noticeable differences in reminiscence between males and females of either of the two age groups. McBride and Payne (1980) write that differences in reminiscence exhibited by males and females on rotary pursuit tasks do not result from innate differences in learning ability, but are due instead to a sex-related capacity for the dissipation of reactive inhibition.

Eysenck and Frith (1977) write that, following rest periods of twenty-four to forty-eight hours, individuals of high ability tend to show higher reminiscence effects in rotary pursuit performance. When there are rest periods of thirty days or longer, subjects of lower ability demonstrated higher levels of reminiscence. Kleinman (1980) studied the effects of distribution of practice and pretask ability on the acquisition of three gymnastic skills and observed no significant differences in the rates of learning between massed and distributed practice groups. Subjects of high ability acquired all the criterion tasks in fewer trials, regardless of the temporal conditions of practice. Interaction between ability and practice condition was observed for only one of the criterion tasks, the glide kip. The acquisition of this task by high-ability subjects was improved by massed practice. Given the inconsistent findings from studies of reminiscence in motor learning, it appears that the interaction between the taxonomy of the task and the individual differences of the learners contributes to determining the effects of distribution of practice in the acquisition of motor skills.

The last area to be dealt with in this chapter is the effortfulness of the experimental task. The assumption is that the more fatiguing the task, the more incremental the effect of distribution of practice. Deese (1958) writes that common opinion expects distribution of practice to be effective for tasks involving a large amount of physical work and effort expenditure. This position, however, was not substantiated by results of studies on gross motor skills (Mohr, 1960). Another refutation of Deese's position is given by Ellis (1953), who writes that Hullian inhibition theory does not permit general predictions of a highly effortful task's effect on reminiscence. Further, a new body of supporting assumptions on how subjects allot energy to the task at hand must be formulated in order to ascertain the degree of independence between the reminiscence phenomenon and the effortfulness of the task.

Eysenck and Frith (1977) contend that physical fatigue can be a major factor in the interaction between level of pretask ability and the conditions of practice. The authors argue that under massed practice, subjects of high ability will make more responses, become more fatigued, and perform at a lower level of proficiency. Since fatigue does not build as readily under distributed practice, subjects of high ability should retain their initial advantage and outperform those of low ability.

### Applications to Teaching

When dealing with the problems of practice distribution within the context of a practical teaching situation, it should be realized that the temporal massing of practice alone may not necessarily result in a performance decrement. Such effects actually accrue from the interaction of a number of complex factors. One is the way in which the learning task itself is paced: externally (by the instructor or by a timing device), or by the subject. The former is far more susceptible to the detrimental effects of massed practice. A student returning balls served by an automatic serving machine is far more likely to be adversely affected by massed practice than one who is simply volleying the ball against a wall for an equal amount of time. Subject-paced tasks are often inherently distributed, regardless of method of practice. The learner performs at a pace he deems most productive, thus precluding the need for distributed practice conditions.

Another factor is the familiarity of the learning task. Students who are learning a skill for the first time will be making many changes and adjustments in their responses. These wide fluctuations in the temporal and spatial application of muscular force tend to "break up" or distribute the practice period even if it is massed. During the acquisition phase, the learner must process information that is highly uncertain. Since such information is low in coherence, $I_R$ can be dissipated even in the absence of a rest period, due to the breaks or inconsistencies in the input signal. Thus, the initial phase of motor learning may be less prone to the adverse effects of massed practice. Conversely, a student performing a task which has been well learned is repeating the exact movements in an identical sequence and is therefore more susceptible to the detrimental effects of massed practice. After the initial acquisition of a task, the learner's responses are successfully adapted to meet the particular requirements governing the temporal and spatial application of muscular force in a highly circumscribed performance situation. When performing an already acquired task, the learner is processing information high in relative redundancy (Kleinman, 1977) and prone to the adverse effects of massed practice.

The nature of the criterion learning task is yet another important factor in determining the effects of practice distribution upon the acquisition of a given skill. Performance upon discrete and continuous tasks rests upon independent and highly task-specific factors. Activities which involve perceptible separations or marked phases in their execution (e.g., foul shooting in basketball, serving in tennis, or putting in golf) tend to be inherently distributed when compared to such continuous tasks as swimming or jogging. Given these differences in taxonomy, it is probable that discrete tasks are less likely to be adversely affected by massing of practice than tasks which are continuous. Therefore, teaching discrete tasks under relatively massed conditions should result in a minimal loss of learning efficiency. In planning an instructional program, it is reasonable, therefore, to assume that discrete activities can be effectively acquired under concentrated practice conditions; continuous skills are best acquired by the temporal distribution of practice.

One must consider, in establishing the temporal patterning of an instructional program of physical activities, the individual differences of the learner. Factors of pretask ability, age, and sex interact significantly with the conditions of practice and the nature of the learning task, but the motivational level of the subjects is important in establishing the temporal patterns of work and rest. Predicated upon the assumption that the detrimental effects of massed practice result from the accumulation of reactive inhibition ($I_R$), the performance of poorly motivated subjects will be susceptible to the adverse effects of massed practice, while highly motivated individuals, such as varsity athletes, will be capable of sustained high levels of performance under intensively massed practice conditions. (Since $I_R$ is a negative drive and motivation a positive one, the higher the subject's motivational level, the greater the resultant tolerance to $I_R$.)

In conclusion, the factors which ultimately determine the most effective temporal distribution of work and rest in a given teaching situation are dependent upon the nature of the criterion task and the individual differences of the learner. There is no general pattern of practice distribution which can ensure maximal rates of acquisition under differing learning conditions. A particular pattern may facilitate performance in a given learning situation, but prove ineffective if any of the conditions of that situation are altered.

### References

Ammons, R.B. "Acquisition of Motor Skill: I. Quantitative Analysis and Theoretical Formulation." *Psychological Review, 54* (1947), 263–281.

————— and, C.H. "Decremental and Related Processes in Skilled Performance." *In* L. E. Smith (ed.), *Psychology of Motor Learning.* Chicago: Athletic Institute, 1970.

Attneave, F. *Applications of Information Theory to Psychology.* New York: Holt, Rinehart and Winston, 1959.

Austin, D.A. "Effects of Distributed and Massed Practice Upon the Learning of a Velocity Task." *Research Quarterly, 46* (1975), 23–30.

Boswell, J.J. and K.C. Spatz. "Reminiscence: A Rich Source of Individual Differences." *Journal of Motor Behavior, 7* (1975), 1–7.

Caron, A.V. "Performance and Learning in a Discrete Motor Task Under Massed vs. Distributed Practice." *Research Quarterly, 40* (1970), 481–489.

Catalano, J.E. "The Effect of Rest Following Massed Practice of

Continuous and Discrete Motor Tasks." *Journal of Motor Behavior, 10* (1978), 63–67.

Cook, B.S. and E.R. Hilgard. "Distributed Practice in Motor Learning." *Journal of Experimental Psychology, 39* (1949), 169–172.

Cook, T.W. "Factors in Massed and Distributed Practice." *Journal of Experimental Psychology, 34,* (1944), 325–334.

Coombs, C.H., R.M. Dawes, and A. Tversky. *Mathematical Psychology.* Englewood Cliffs, NJ: Prentice-Hall, 1970.

Deese, J. *The Psychology of Learning.* New York: McGraw-Hill, 1958.

Dore, L. and E.R. Hilgard. "Spaced Practice and the Maturation Hypothesis." *Journal of Psychology, 4* (1937), 245–259.

————. "Spaced Practice As a Test of Snoddy's Two Processes in Mental Growth." *Journal of Experimental Psychology, 23* (1938) , 359–374.

Duncan, C.P. "The Effects of Unequal Amounts of Practice on Motor Learning Before and After Rest." *Journal of Experimental Psychology,* 42 (1951), 257–264.

Ellis, D.S. "Inhibition Theory and the Effort Variable." *Psychological Review, 60* (1953), 383–392.

Eysenck, H.J. "An Experimental Test of the Inhibition and Consolidation Theories of Reminiscence." *Life Sciences, 3* (1964), 175 – 188.

————. "A Three Factor Theory of Reminiscence." *British Journal of Psychology, 56* (1965), 168–181.

———— and C. D. Frith. *Reminiscence, Motivation and Personality.* New York: Plenum Press, 1977.

Fitts, P.M. "Factors in Complex Skill Training." *In* R. Glaser (ed.), *Training Research and Education.* Pittsburgh: Pittsburgh University Press, 1962.

————. "Perceptual-Motor Skill Learning." *In* A.W. Melton (ed.), *Categories of Human Learning.* New York: Academic Press, 1964.

Fleishman, E.A. "Abilities at Different Stages of Practice in Rotary Pursuit Performance." *Journal of Experimental Psychology, 60* (1960), 162–171.

————. *The Structure and Measurement of Physical Fitness.* Englewood Cliffs, NJ.: Prentice-Hall, 1964.

————. "Human Abilities and the Acquisition of Skill." *In* E.A. Bilodeau (ed.), *Acquisition of Skill.* New York: Academic Press, 1966.

————. "Individual Differences and Motor Learning." *In* R.M. Gagné (ed.), *Learning and Individual Differences.* Columbus, Ohio: Merrill, 1967.

Franklin, J.C. and J. Brozek. "The Relation Between Distribution of

Practice and Learning Efficiency in Psychomotor Performance." *Journal of Experimental Psychology, 37* (1947), 16–24.

Gagné, R.M. and E.A. Fleishman. *Psychology and Human Performance.* New York: Henry Holt. 1959.

Harmon, J.M. and J.B. Crendine. "Effects of Different Lengths of Practice Periods on the Learning of a Motor Skill." *Research Quarterly, 32* (1961), 34–41.

————— and A.P. Miller. "Time Patterns in Motor Learning." *Research Quarterly, 21* (1950), 182–187.

Hsu, S.H. and R.B. Payne. "Effector Localization and Transfer of Reactive Inhibition." *Journal of Motor Behavior, 11* (1979), 153–158.

Huang, K.L. and R.B. Payne. "Transfer of Reactive Inhibition." *Journal of Motor Behavior, 9* (1977), 293–300.

Hull, C.L. *A Behavior System: An Introduction to Behavior Theory Concerning the Individual Organism.* New Haven, Conn.: Yale University Press, 1952.

Irion, A.L. "Reminiscence and Warm Up." *In* L. M. Stolurow (ed.), *Readings in Learning.* New York: Prentice-Hall, 1953.

—————. "A Brief History of Research on the Acquisition of Skill." In E.A. Bilodeau (ed.), *Acquisition of Skill.* New York: Academic Press, 1966.

Kintsch, W. *Learning, Memory and Conceptual Processes.* New York: John Wiley, 1970.

Kleinman, M. "The Effects of Practice Distribution on the Acquisition of Three Discrete Motor Skills." *Research Quarterly, 47* (1976), 672–677.

—————. "Ability Factors in Motor Learning." *Perceptual and Motor Skills, 44* (1977), 827–836.

—————. "Distribution of Practice and Pre-Task Ability in the Acquisition of Three Discrete Gross Motor Skills." *Perceptual and Motor Skills, 51* (1980), 935–944.

Knapp, B. *Skill in Sport: The Attainment of Proficiency.* London: Routledge and Kegan Paul, 1966.

Knapp, C. and R. Dixon. "Learning to Juggle: I. A Study to Determine the Effects of Two Different Distributions of Practice on Learning and Efficiency." *Research Quarterly, 21* (1950), 331–336.

McBride, D.K. and R.B. Payne. "Psychomotor Reminiscence As a Function of Sex and Length of Rest Period." *Journal of Motor Behavior, 11* (1979), 59–64.

—————. "The Sex Difference in Rotary Pursuit: Aptitude or Inhibition?" *Journal of Motor Behavior, 12* (1980), 270–280.

McGeoch, J.A. and A.L. Irion. *The Psychology of Human Learning.* New York: McKay, 1961.

Mohr, D. R. "The Contributions of Physical Activity to Skill Learning." *Research Quarterly, 31* (1960), 321–350.

Noble, C.E. "Age, Race, and Sex in the Learning and Performance of Psychomotor Skills" *In* T. Osborne, C. Noble, and N. Weyl (eds.), *Human Variation: The Biopsychology of Age, Race, and Sex.* New York: Academic Press, 1978.

_____, O.G. Salazar, C.S. Skelley, and R. H. Wilkerson. "Work and Rest Variables in the Acquisition of Psychomotor Tracking Skill." *Journal of Motor Behavior, 11* (1979), 233–246.

Payne, R.B. and K.L. Huang. "Interaction of Sex and Task Differences in Reminiscence." *Journal of Motor Behavior, 9* (1977), 29–32.

Purohit, A.P. "Massed Practice in Pursuit Rotor Tasks and Two Factor Theory of Inhibition."*Journal of General Psychology, 78* (1968), 9–17.

Richardson, A. "Mental Practice: A Review and Discussion." *In* R.N. Singer (ed.), *Readings in Motor Learning.* Philadelphia: Lea and Febiger, 1972.

Singer, R.N. "Massed and Distributed Practice Effects on the Acquisition and Retention of a Novel Basketball Skill." *Research Quarterly, 36* (1965), 68–77.

Smith, K.U. "Cybernetic Theory and Analysis of Learning." In E.A. Bilodeau (ed.), *Acquisition of Skill.* New York: Academic Press, 1966.

_____ and M.F. *Cybernetic Principles of Learning and Educational Design.* New York: Holt, Rinehart and Winston, 1966.

Stelmach, G.E. "Distribution of Practice in Individual Differences and Intra-Variability." *Perceptual and Motor Skills, 26* (1968), 727–730.

Travis, R.C. "Practice and Rest Periods in Motor Learning." *Journal of Psychology, 3* (1936), 183–187.

Young, O.C. "Rate of Learning in Relation to Spacing of Practice Periods in Archery and Badminton." *Research Quarterly, 25* (1954), 231–243.

# PART II

Learning As Information Processing

# CHAPTER 6

# Neurophysiological Factors in Motor Learning

MOTOR LEARNING RESEARCH during the past half century has been dominated by a decidedly behavioristic approach in terms of its philosophical and methodological orientation. The learner is treated as a passive entity whose behavior is determined solely by the manipulation of such environmental variables as number of reinforcements, serial order of learning, or temporal distribution of work and rest. Unfortunately, this approach has failed to account satisfactorily for the interaction between the nature of the learning task and the individual differences of the learner. This interaction is fundamental to the acquisition and performance of purposive, goal-directed, complex motor skills. Improved knowledge of the neurophysiological mechanisms which underlie motor control will yield insight into the nature of the specific information-processing capacities necessary to the acquisition and performance of complex motor activities. With such knowledge, the researcher can better control environmental variables and predict their interaction with factors related to individual differences.

The acquisition of motor skill is a dynamic process involving interaction between the learner and the environment, mediated through the integration of reflexive and voluntary neurological activity. Stimulus information, or environmental input, is conveyed through afferent pathways to central association areas where appropriate responses are effected and consequently manifested in the form of behavioral output. In addition to attempting to accomplish a purpose or goal, a movement alters the environment, consequently affecting the input to the learner. The response of a tennis player striking the ball with a racket not only accomplishes the goal of returning the opponent's shot, but also alters the entire pattern of a stimulus input. In fact, the response would alter the environment (change the position of the racket, in this case), whether or not the goal of the movement is fulfilled. The afferent input from the altered stimulus situation provides the learner with necessary information feedback to adjust and modify the response pattern further. The greater the complexity of the response, the greater the need for dynamic interaction between the learner and the environment. The nervous system, therefore, regulates and controls the continuous series of changes and adjustments which characterize complex motor activity.

The nervous system serves as the link between physical reality and subjective experience. It is the biological mechanism allowing an individual to translate thought into action. It is the physical substrate of such complex behavioral phenomena as learning, memory, and even consciousness itself. In order to regulate and control these activities precisely, the nervous system must continually process a stream of afferent input which conveys coded information about the conditions prevailing in the external world. Although there are many forms of afferent information impinging upon an individual at any one time, only a fraction of this input gives rise to conscious experience and is defined as sensory information. Once it is internalized, the coded afferent input differs greatly from the actual conditions (sound, light, motion) which it represents. It conveys information on the intensity, quality, duration, and location of a given stimulus.

The regulation of movement requires the synergistic action of groups of neurons firing in parallel. Although this replication of function appears superficially to be wasteful, it is due precisely to these high levels of redundancy that one can achieve the degree of accuracy and consistency associated with motor output. A pattern of movement depends upon the number of nerves that fire or remain silent at a particular temporal moment. If one were dealing with a hypothetical nerve net consisting of three neurons, there would be $2^3$ or 8 possible combinations in which those three nerves could fire. (See Figure 6-1) Since any neuron can exhibit only one of two possible conditions (on or off), the nervous system clearly functions on a binary basis in which the number of possible outcomes is calculated by raising the base 2 to a power predicated upon the number of nerves involved. For example, a nerve net consisting of 10 neurons would result in $2^{10}$ or 1,024 possible combinations.

The question often arises how the all-or-none function of a neuron can result in the complexities of human behavior. Since a neuron cannot modulate its output—it either fires or remains silent—information is transmitted in the nervous system through a binary code based upon the temporal patterning of the sequence of impulses along the membrane of a given nerve. Unlike a wire, a neuron does not conduct impulses in direct proportion to the strength with which they are generated. The impulse is transmitted along the membrane as a wave of excitation. Each wave or "spike" is of uniform amplitude, regardless of the intensity of the stimulus. The frequency of these waves conveys the strength or weakness of the stimulus: the closer the spikes, the greater the intensity of the stimulus; the greater the spacing between the spikes, the weaker the stimulus. (See Figure 6-2)

**Figure 6-1**

## POSSIBLE COMBINATIONS IN 3-NEURON NETWORK

| combination | neuron 1 | neuron 2 | neuron 3 |
|:---:|:---:|:---:|:---:|
| 1 | x | x | x |
| 2 | o | o | o |
| 3 | x | x | o |
| 4 | o | o | x |
| 5 | o | x | o |
| 6 | x | o | x |
| 7 | x | o | o |
| 8 | o | x | x |

x = on
o = off

**Figure 6-2**

## STIMULUS INTENSITY AND
## ACTION POTENTIAL FREQUENCY

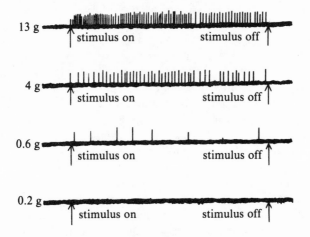

Action potentials in a single afferent nerve fiber in response to the application of various constant-pressure stimuli to the mechanosensitive receptor ending.

Although the mechanisms underlying the firing of a neuron are extremely complex, the action potential or spike depends upon a difference in electrical charge between the inside and the outside of the membrane.* There can be no neurological activity unless this difference in membrane potential is present. The action potential is actually a wave of excitation which proceeds along the membrane by causing the section of the membrane immediately following the spike to depolarize. The minimal amount of stimulation necessary to elicit an action potential is known as the neural threshold. Following the action potential, there is a brief period known as the absolute refractory phase when no amount of stimulation will cause a neuron to fire. This is followed by the relative refractory period in which the neuron may be stimulated to fire if, and only if, the stimulus is greater than that normally required to activate it. In effect, during the relative refractory period, the threshold becomes elevated. It is seen that an inverse relationship exists between the threshold of a neuron and its sensitivity: the higher the sensitivity, the lower the threshold; the lower the sensitivity, the higher the threshold.

In contrast to the all-or-none property of the action potential, specialized receptors which respond to external stimuli generate a graded potential which varies in its frequency as well as its amplitude. Such a graded or receptor potential has neither a threshold nor a refractory period. It is capable of the summation of impulses, i.e., several weak stimuli occurring within close temporal proximity will exert a cumulative effect upon its amplitude. The greater the number and intensity of the stimuli impinging upon the receptor, the greater the frequency and the amplitude of the receptor potential. If the resultant receptor potential is sufficiently strong to exceed the threshold of an afferent neuron, a chain of action potentials will result whose frequency will be in direct proportion to the intensity of the receptor potential.

The binary nature of the action potential provides the mechanism for transforming the analog signal of the receptor into the digitized signal of the afferent neuronal pathway. This analog to digital conversion in turn provides the means for conveying large amounts of information with maximal accuracy. (A digitized signal is far less prone to distortion during the course of its transmission than an analog signal.) This binary code is the internal language of the nervous system and enables the organism to elicit rapid and accurate responses to changing environmental stimuli.

Relating neurological activity to purposive motor behavior, one finds an ever-increasing pattern of complexity in motor activity which

---

*In the resting state, the outside is positively charged and the inside is negatively charged.

parallels the organization of the motor system itself. The basic element of goal-directed motor patterns is the reflex. Sherrington (1948) argues that the most highly developed level of neural function is found in the regulation and control of motor activity. He asserts that the study of reflexive activity can provide a knowledge of the basic integrative mechanisms which function in the absence of cognitive involvement. The role of individual reflexes diminishes and higher-order integrative activity becomes more important as the organism becomes more biologically complex.

Sherrington refers to reflexive activity as behavior which is essentially controlled by innate biological circuitry rather than by learning. The reflex accounts for the motor mechanism in animals which can be elicited in the absence of cognitive involvement. (A dog perks up its ears in response to a sound, even though it lacks insight into the purpose of this activity.) Specialized nerve receptors analyze the successive situations occurring between the organism and the environment. A reflex is defined as an animal's reaction to the surrounding environment. Changes in the environment result in corresponding changes in muscular involvement and reflexive patterns of movement, so that a series of motor acts results from a corresponding series of successive external situations. Sherrington argues that the nervous system functions as an integrative system through reflex action. One of its primary functions is the translation of external sensory information into sensation and ideation. From a purely philosophical viewpoint, the nervous system is the integrative element of the mind and the body.

Nerves have the power to transmit spatially (conduct) states of excitement (nerve impulses) which are generated by specialized receptors. The neuronal integration of the external and internal environment coordinates the life processes throughout the organism in a relatively efficient manner. At least three distinct structures comprise reflexive integration: 1) an effector organ, such as a muscle or gland; 2) a conducting nervous pathway leading to the effector organ; and 3) an initiating organ or receptor where the the reaction starts. This entire system is classified as a reflex arc. (See Figure 6-3) That part of the system leading up to but not including the effector is called the afferent arc. If the nervous system is studied from the standpoint of its integrative activity, the reflex arc is the fundamental unit mechanism of neuronal activity. However, not every reflex constitutes a unit action. There are many reflex activities (e.g., walking) which require the compounding of a number of simple reflexes. Some contemporary theorists view the early phases of child development in these terms. The concept of the simple reflex may well be an abstraction rather than reality. All parts of the nervous system are interconnected: neither can a single segment act alone, nor can any part ever be completely at rest.

## Figure 6-3

## DIAGRAM OF A SIMPLE REFLEX ARC

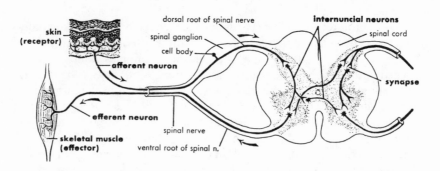

According to Sherrington, the basis of nervous coordination lies in the compounding of reflexes. There are two grades of reflexive coordination: the simple reflex itself, and the coordination and interaction among several reflexes. Such coordination entails the orderly coadjustment of several synchronous reflexes, a process which may well explain one of the major physiological bases of motor learning. This orderly succession of responses involves the suppression or inhibition of one reflex by another or one group of reflexes by another group, and is characterized by the orderly change from one reflex pattern of behavior to another. For this succession to occur in an orderly manner, no inharmonious component of the previous reflex may remain. If, for example, the new response involves the activity of extensor muscles, as in throwing or striking, the antagonistic activity of the flexor muscles must be inhibited. When the change from one reflex to another occurs, it is therefore usually far-reaching and spread over a wide range of nervous arcs. Much of coordinated, goal-directed motor behavior is dependent upon the complex interactions of such compound reflex patterns.

Motor activity is regulated by two functional divisions of the nervous system: the pyramidal and the extrapyramidal motor systems. The pyramidal motor system primarily covers the initiation of voluntary movement; the extrapyramidal system, its regulation and control. The pyramidal system is comprised of the pyramidal tract, which originates in the main motor area of the cerebral cortex and innervates individual or small groups of muscles. In contrast, the extrapyramidal system is comprised of several parts of the brain, including the cerebellum, the thalamus, the basal ganglia, and the brain stem. Its primary function is regulation and control of movement based upon proprioceptive or kinesthetic information relating to the acceleration and displacement of the various body segments. (See Figure 6-4)

## Figure 6-4

## A SIMPLIFIED SCHEMA OF THE MOTOR SYSTEM

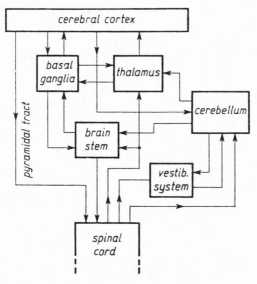

### Cortical Control

Although basic movements are regulated reflexively, the execution of coordinated, integrated patterns of movement requires cortical involvement. The cerebral cortex has three basic functions: afferent, which involves the processing of sensory information; efferent, which involves the elicitation of motor responses; and associative, critical in the mediation of complex behavior, which involves the processing of sensory and motor information. It is the latter which constitutes the physical basis for the translation of sensation into action. Motor activities requiring precise control (e.g., fine manipulative skills) are under the control of the cerebral cortex. The greater the degree of precision required in a movement, the greater the extent to which cortical mechanisms will be called in to override the muscular set, which is autonomically established by brain stem mechanisms.* The main motor area of the cerebral cortex consists of colonies of giant pyramidal cells. Through the use of microelectronic techniques, it has been observed that stimulation of individual cells results in the activation of particular muscles. It is reasoned, therefore, that each cell represents a single motor unit in a particular muscle.

A motor unit consists of a single motor axon (nerve fiber) and a group of muscle cells which are all innervated by that one fiber. (See Figure 6-5) Each motor unit functions in an all-or-none (binary) fashion, i.e., all the muscle cells in a given unit are in a state of contraction or relaxation at any one point in time. (There are no intermediate states of activity.) The size of a motor unit can vary from five to seven cells per axon (as in the muscles of the fingers) to as many as 2,000 cells per axon (as in the large antigravity muscles). The greater the number of motor units in a given muscle, the greater the degree of control which can be exerted over it. Muscles requiring precise control have a high number of small motor units; muscles requiring a grosser form of control have a relatively small number of large motor units. Muscular force is modulated through the coordinated activity of the motor units within a given muscle. A large number of motor units are recruited when a great deal of force is needed, a small number, when the action requires only minimal force.

On the other hand, coordinated muscular activity is based upon the temporal sequencing (timing) of the firing pattern of the motor units. This synergistic activity is a prime physiological factor in motor learning. As proficiency develops, the learner becomes capable of exerting precise control over the individual motor unit's temporal duration of activity. In a highly skilled individual, this regulatory process is initiated volitionally, but carried out in an automated fashion below the level of consciousness. The degree of precise control an individual is capable of exerting in the performance of a motor task is directly related to the coordinated functioning of the motor units in the involved muscles. The greater the degree of control exerted over a given muscle, the greater the number of motor units as well as degree of cortical representation (the higher the number of pyramidal cells representing that particular muscle). (See Figure 6-6) The stimulation of a given pyramidal cell will always result in the activation of the same motor unit in the same muscle. It is through the integration of afferent

---

*Brain stem mechanisms control many motor activities, particularly maintenance of posture. The need to override a muscular set is most noticeable in movements involving the antigravity muscles.

### Figure 6-5

## MOTOR UNIT ORGANIZATION

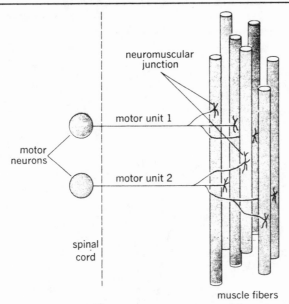

Muscle fibers associated with two motor neurons, forming two motor units within a muscle.

information that the cortex can elicit the appropriate muscular responses required in the execution of a complex act.

According to Brooks (1969), voluntary movement is initiated in the motor area of the cerebral cortex and regulated through the processing of kinesthetic and somatosensory feedback information by specialized cortical association areas. Sensations such as pain, pressure, heat, and cold are processed within the primary sensory area of the cortex, and information pertaining to the static state of muscles is processed by sensory areas within the motor cortex itself. However, information concerning dynamic factors, such as the degree of change in muscle length or the velocity of contraction, is channeled to a narrow strip between the motor area and the sensory area of the cortex. The motor cortex processes information relating to the external and internal environment. Peripheral information from auditory and visual afferents is relayed to the motor cortex through lower brain centers.* Knowledge

---

*There appear to be no direct cortical connections between the visual and auditory association areas and the motor area.

**Figure 6-6**

## DIAGRAM OF THE DIRECT CORTICOSPINAL PATHWAY

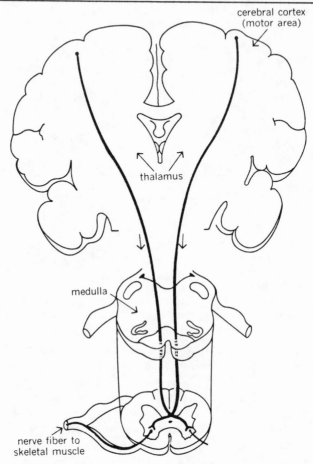

cerebral cortex
(motor area)

thalamus

medulla

nerve fiber to
skeletal muscle

of body orientation in space converges through the vestibular system. However, the main afferent information entering the motor cortex is in the form of exteroceptive input from the skin and proprioceptive input from the tendons and muscles. Unfortunately, little is known about the cortical integration of kinesthetic information.

Maiorov et al. (1980) write that although much of the motor command content sent from the cortex to the peripheral effector mechanisms (the muscles) has been determined, the influence of sensory feedback upon the processes forming these cortical motor commands is still unclear. The authors contend that afferent signals from the involved limb segments exert a positive feedback effect which is vital to the formation and the initiation of the cortical motor command. Glencross and Koreman (1979) argue that the initiation and control of movement is dependent upon a series of peripheral feedback loops which serve in the preservation and the processing of afferent information. This afferent feedback functions as an orienting or attentional mechanism which precisely focuses and refines the output of the motor cortex.

There is still controversy about the role of the motor cortex in the execution and control of movement. A central issue is the extent to which it actually initiates rather than merely regulates and controls movement through the processing of sensory feedback information. Evarts (1967), for example, questions whether the primary output variable of the motor cortex pertains to the direction and extent of movement or to the forces underlying the movement. Based upon empirical observation, Evarts contends that the relative importance of force, duration, and direction in the control of motor activity varies from movement to movement, and that all voluntary movement depends upon the cooperative actions of these three factors.

This discussion aside, there is also the question of the organization of the motor cortex itself. Is the central factor the control of individual muscles, or the regulation of entire patterns of movement? Evarts argues that cortical organization is differentiated into specialized areas which respond to changes in muscular force and limb displacement, as well as areas which control individual muscles and regulate whole patterns of movement. Muscles are not represented in the cerebral cortex according to size. The areas of the body where skill and finesse of movement are most important, such as the thumb, tongue, lips, and larynx, are represented over the largest areas of the motor cortex by pyramidal cells arranged in specific colonies. According to Eccles (1973), each colony embodies a column of pyramidal cells representing the various motor units in a given muscle. Although each colony represents a different muscle, colonies representing muscles engaged in a common activity (e.g., flexion of the thumb) lie in close proximity to one another in the motor cortex.

Current evidence indicates, therefore, that muscles as well as movements are represented in the cortex. Contrary to the arguments of J. H. Jackson,* however, each muscle is represented only one time. There is a direct relationship between the number of motor units in a given muscle and the degree of representation that muscle is allotted in the cerebral cortex: those muscles requiring the greatest degree of

---

*Jackson thought that each muscle is represented many times over in different parts of the motor cortex, each part concerned with the execution of specific movement patterns.

control are given the largest representation; those requiring only gross regulation are given minimal representation. (See Figure 6-7)

**Figure 6-7**

## MOTOR AREAS OF THE CEREBRAL CORTEX

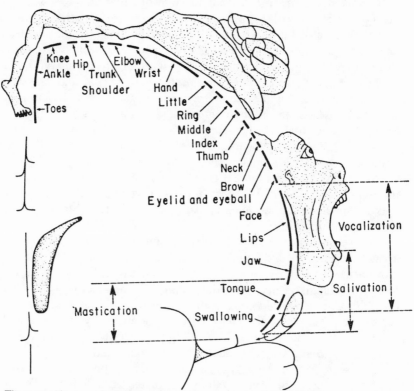

The motor "homunculus" of the precentral area: a coronal section of the precentral gyrus and the location of the motor cortical representation of different parts of the body. The size of the various parts is proportional to the amount of cortical surface area serving them.

Luria (1966) writes that the direction and coordination of voluntary movement depends upon the integrative functions of higher-order centers of the cerebral cortex. The giant pyramidal (Betz) cells are merely trigger mechanisms governing the specific exit point for nerve impulses traveling from the motor cortex to a given muscle. Luria's stand is that coordinated motor activity depends entirely upon the capacity of the cortex to analyze proprioceptive and exteroceptive information feedback arising from the movements of the learner himself.

It is precisely through this cortical analysis of the information feedback emanating from the involved body segments that the entire course of a complex motor activity is continually monitored and regulated.

Luria argues that the integrative mechanisms governing the execution of coordinated patterns of movement—throwing, jumping, running—are not inherent in the structural organization of the centers which effect movement (the Betz cells), but lie instead in the plasticity of the cortex itself. The cortex is not arranged in terms of specific areas, preprogramed to execute stereotyped patterns of response, but is instead a complex integrative mechanism which synthesizes sensory input, reflexive activity, and conscious, purposive, goal-directed behavior. It is the capacity of the cortex to integrate and synthesize the afferent (feedback) information systematically that provides the framework for the precise organization and coordination of complex movement. The Betz cells represent specific muscles, just as the keys of a piano represent musical notes. Just as striking the keys in a given sequence results in a particular melody, the excitation of specific Betz cells by higher centers of the cerebral cortex results in particular movement patterns.

Luria substantiates his position by citing anatomical evidence which indicates that as the phylogenetic complexity of an organism increases, the volume of Betz cells decreases in relation to the volume of the controlling afferent apparatus. There are, for example, more Betz cells found in the cortex of a monkey than in the human motor cortex, but the human cells are larger. In addition to the difference in size, each Betz cell in the human receives a greater number of afferent synaptic inputs. It is this increase in afferent input that enables humans to manifest such a wide range of motor skills and to exert such precise levels of motor control.

Luria's arguments on the central role of cortical integration in the performance of complex motor activities is substantiated by Eccles (1973), who cites evidence indicating that voluntary movement is preceded by a readiness potential which is recorded from the association areas of the cortex. The readiness potential precedes a movement by as much as .8 seconds and is believed to represent the communication between the major and minor cortical hemispheres during the selection and programing of a given movement. Eccles contends that the readiness potential is evidence of the neurological activity underlying the transmission of ideation into movement. Although the precise mechanisms are not fully understood, motor activity is apparently initiated by specific excitation of the motor cortex, which is preceded by a nonspecific or general excitation over the cortical areas associated with thought and reasoning. In effect, it is within the cerebral cortex that the desire to execute a particular movement is translated into action.

The structure of the cerebral cortex may give some clue to the role it plays in motor learning. The cortex is divided into two hemispheres: the major or dominant, and the minor or nondominant. In 98 percent of cases, regardless of handedness, the left hemisphere is dominant and the right nondominant. (See Figure 6-8)

The stage of development in which hemispheric specialization occurs is undecided. Kaufman et al. (1978) write that the precise relationship of lateral dominance (hand, foot, or eye) to lateral cerebral specialization and interhemispheric integration is not clearly understood. However, relationships were observed between hand dominance and such factors as left-right awareness, mental ability, and motor coordination for normal preschool and elementary school children. The authors saw that children who established hand dominance at a young age (2½ to 4½) demonstrated higher levels of intelligence and better coordination. Turkewitz (1977) argues that the brain actually becomes laterally differentiated during early infancy. He feels that the brain's capacity to manifest a compensatory function (e.g., the mediation of speech by centers in the minor hemisphere) in response to an injury during the early years of childhood describes its inherent plasticity.

The relationship between an individual's sex and the degree of hemispheric differentiation is also argued. McGlone (1980) writes that there is a significant body of evidence indicating that the male brain may be more asymmetrically organized than the brain of the female, both for verbal and nonverbal functions. (Males tend to perform better on spatial tasks; females, on verbal tasks.) The author contends that these trends are rarely found in childhood but become increasingly significant as the individual matures.

Eccles (1977) further states that cortical hemispheres possess complementary functions which facilitate the processing of specific types of information and the integration of ideational and motoric activities. An analogy may be drawn between the structure of the cerebral cortex and the function of a hybrid computer in which half the device handles analog data and the other half processes digital data. The nondominant hemisphere is like an analog computer; it processes temporal and spatial data as opposed to abstract information. The major hemisphere resembles a digital computer; it deals with abstract or digital information. Although both hemispheres are in continual communication, many of the events experienced by the nondominant hemisphere cannot be verbalized by the major hemisphere. This is particularly true when one is confronted with the need to verbalize a motor skill. It is difficult to express with verbal accuracy the temporal and spatial elements which constitute the execution of a motor skill.

## Figure 6-8

## DOMINANT AND NONDOMINANT CORTICAL HEMISPHERES

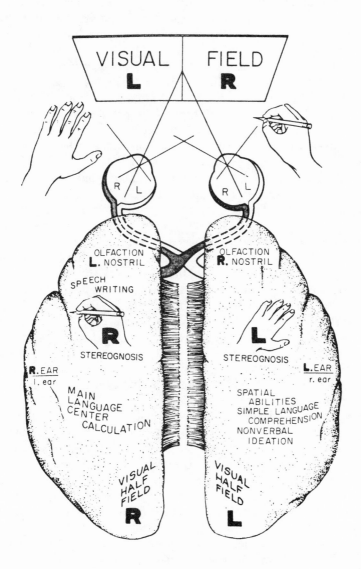

Functions separated by surgery. A simplified summary combined from known neuroanatomy, cortical lesion data, and postoperative testing.

The nondominant hemisphere is the conscious link with the reflexive control mechanisms of motor learning. Proprioceptive feedback is integrated with visual input here and the appropriate adjustments are effected. Since a motor skill involves the precise temporal and spatial application of varying amounts of force, the minor hemisphere is all-important in the conscious mediation of motor activities. Striking a moving ball with a bat or a racket, catching a running pass, or "getting the jump" on a fly ball are examples of situations in which the minor hemisphere plays an essential role. The minor hemisphere deals with physical events in time and space rather than with abstractions; its language is speed, force, time, and direction. Understanding the principles, rules, and strategies of a skill are processing functions of the major cortical hemisphere. The actual execution of the skill comes from nonverbal information processed in the nondominant hemisphere. The interaction between the two in motor learning is not fully understood.

The complex nature of the initiation of voluntary movement is further described by Eyzaguirre and Fidone (1975). The authors write that stimulation of pyramidal tract fibers resulted in evoked excitatory potentials in the frontal and parietal lobes of the cerebral cortex. (Both these areas are involved in associative processes.) These findings, they say, indicate that a large part of the major motor pathway arises in the nonmotor cortex. The Betz cells of the motor area, therefore, are not the sole source of origin of the pyramidal tract. Just as the pyramidal tract arises from diverse origins within the cortex, it also terminates upon diverse structures within the spinal cord. The influence of the pyramidal tract is not confined merely to skeletomotor and fusimotor neurons, but extends to the interneurons which control proprioceptive and extero-ceptive sensory inflow. In addition to innervating specific muscles, the efferent discharge of the pyramidal tract modifies afferent input through the mechanism of presynaptic inhibition.

Given this arrangement, even in the case of pyramidal discharge (a phenomenon characteristically regarded as purely efferent), there is a direct effect upon afferent input. Such effects, however, are confined to facilitating the two basic functions of the pyramidal system: initiating volitional control of movement and overcoming the reflexively controlled postural set of the muscles involved in the movement. The greater the dexterity required in a muscular movement, the greater the pyramidal facilitation of the involved muscle. Conversely, the greater the role of a muscle in the maintenance of posture (primarily in terms of the degree to which it exerts an antigravity function), the greater the pyramidal inhibition of that muscle.

Although the motor cortex functions as a highly complex integrative mechanism, reciprocal innervation of antagonistic muscles does not appear to be an inherent property of cerebral motor unit organization. The excitation of a cortical column which causes a given muscle to contract does not necessarily simultaneously elicit the inhibition of the antagonistic muscle. But coordinated movement depends upon alternating patterns of contraction and relaxation, i.e., excitatory innervation of one group of muscles must be accompanied by inhibitory stimulation of the antagonistic group. Eyzaguirre and Fidone write that the execution of coordinated patterns of volitional movement in humans stems from peripheral afferent input which is processed through preprogramed reciprocal circuits within the spinal cord. The implications of these findings to motor learning are clear. Despite the central role of the cerebral cortex in the initiation and control of volitional activities, the acquisition and performance of motor skills is greatly dependent upon peripheral feedback.

### The Cerebellum

The cerebellum is essential in the subconscious mediation of movement, particularly highly speeded movements such as athletic skills. According to Eccles (1973), the cerebellum functions as a type of in-line computer system concerned with the smooth and efficient regulation of movement. Eccles et al. (1967) describe the cerebellum as a relatively simple neuronal machine which is organized in a precise geometric pattern (a rectangular laminated lattice) uniform throughout the cerebellar cortex. It processes input information in a preprogramed, stereotyped fashion. The cerebellar cortex consists of three layers:

1.  The outermost or molecular, which contains cell bodies of only two types of neurons, basket cells and stellate cells, both of which are confined to this layer only.
2.  The ganglionic, which contains the bodies of Purkinje cells, ascending dendrites of Golgi cells, and several ascending axons.
3.  The granular, which is densely packed with granule neurons and contains Golgi cells, as well as axons which are ascending to or descending from upper layers.

There are three neuronal pathways associated with the flow of information into and out of the cerebellum: the mossy fibers (which anatomists call MF), the climbing fibers (CF), and the axons of Purkinje cells (PC). All cerebellar input (afferent information) is conveyed along the climbing fibers and the mossy fibers, and all cerebellar output (efferent information) along the Purkinje cell fibers. Both afferent pathways convey input from essentially the same peripheral sources (receptors in skin, joint, muscle, and fascia), but differ markedly in the manner in which they transmit their input to the Purkinje cells and in the effects they exert upon them.

Each Purkinje cell receives its input from a single climbing fiber. The mossy fiber input is characterized by extreme convergence, in that a single Purkinje cell may receive information from as many as 80,000 synaptic inputs. In addition to the diversity in the nature of their respective inputs to the Purkinje cells, the mossy fiber and climbing fiber pathways manifest functional differences. The former exerts an inhibitory effect (through basket cells) and an excitatory effect (through granule cells); the latter exerts solely an excitatory effect (through granule cells). Excitatory stimulation of Purkinje cells results in increased inhibitory output. Inhibitory stimulation, in contrast, decreases this output. The net effect of the latter condition is the disinhibition of the target neurons of the Purkinje cells (the four cerebellar nuclei).

The inhibitory action of the Purkinje cells is exerted upon neurons which continually manifest strong excitatory background activity. This activity must be overcome in order to shape and control complex, goal-directed patterns of movement precisely. Purkinje cells which share similar cutaneous and muscular afferent inputs (receive information from the same body segment) tend to be arranged in colonies. Their output is marked by a high degree of convergence upon common target neurons. Although the apparent redundancy in Purkinje output may seem wasteful, it ensures that cerebellar commands will be precisely executed. The colony arrangement also facilitates the organized processing of input data, further enhancing the specificity and precision of cerebellar output. Eccles (1969) writes that there is probably little communication between these colonies or zones because the association pathways within the cerebellum are inhibitory.

Eccles (1973) contends that all cerebellar input is ultimately trans-formed into inhibitory action.* This inhibitory dominance is of great value in the computer-like operation of the cerebellum, particularly related to the execution of highly speeded movements. Whereas chains of excitatory neurons would result in prolonged activity or after-discharge long after the cessation of a given message, the inhibitory action of the cerebellum results in an automatic "cleansing action." In as little as .1 second, a given area of the cerebellum can be cleared and made ready for the next computation. There is constant interaction between excitatory and inhibitory impulses. Thus, no excitatory input can freely exert its effect upon a Purkinje cell, regardless of its intensity.

---

*With the exception of the granule cells, all neurons in the cerebellar cortex exert an inhibitory effect.

It is this constant interaction which results in a continually variable cerebellar output and provides the physical basis for the computer-like operation of the cerebellum.

The cerebellum is linked to the spinal cord and the cerebral cortex through a system of dynamic loops. Its basic function is that of a comparator. It receives an exact copy of the output of the motor cortex as it is being conveyed to the muscles through the motoneurons, detects variations in this information, and effects the necessary corrections. In addition to its role in the monitoring and "fine tuning" of cortical output, the cerebellum is the primary center for the processing of proprioceptive information. Since the cerebellum occupies a position that allows it to compare the output of the motor cortex with the actual outcome of those commands, it is able continually to adjust and refine this output according to proprioceptive information feedback. The cerebellum minimizes the discrepancy between the response desired and the one actually attained. Although the cerebellum is far more limited in its associative functions than the cerebral cortex, it is capable of effecting more rapid corrections, an attribute which makes it a critical adjunct to the acquisition and performance of highly speeded motor activities.

According to Eccles' dynamic loop hypothesis, the upper loop or cerebro-cerebellar pathway enables the cerebellum to provide for extremely rapid correction of evolving movements, i.e., all movements initiated by the motor cortex are almost instantaneously corrected by the cerebellum as they evolve.* The motor cortex alters its output in response to the cerebellar correction. The corrected output is, in turn, further refined by the action of the cerebellum. The return circuit arrangement is believed to underlie the control of all voluntary movement.

The cerebellum regulates movement at subconscious levels by processing afferent information generated by muscle and joint proprioceptors through a more simplified version of the dynamic loop. These spino-cerebellar or lower loop connections operate in walking, standing, balancing, and in all postural adjustments related to active movement. Proprioceptive information is relayed to the cerebellum through the spino-cerebellar tract and from there, following adjustment, down to motoneurons through the vestibulo-spinal tract. Proprioceptive infor-

---

*The time needed to process information feedback in the cerebro-cerebellar pathway is estimated to be about 20msc. (milliseconds) or 1/50 of a second, while processing time in the spino-cerebellar or lower loop is estimated to range between 100 to 200 msc., or between 1/10 and 1/5 of a second.

mation conveyed by the lower loop also supports the programing of the cerebellum. This feedback information is stored and employed as a model or template against which feedback from succeeding responses can be compared. Once it has been programed, the cerebellum can function as a repository of motor information, expediting the execution of complex patterns of movement.

The cerebellar cortex is believed to contain great storage capacity for this information. The cortex of the cerebellum is divided into various subsets. Each individual subset integrates its own particular inputs of information. How these various cerebellar subsets are themselves integrated remains a largely unanswered question. Since there is apparently no communication among the subsets—each one functions more or less independently—it is clear that the overall integration of cerebellar activity is dependent upon factors lying outside the cerebellum. Eccles (1969) contends that the integrative mechanism of the cerebellum lies in the cerebro-cortical and the cerebro-spinal dynamic loops. He believes that feedback from peripheral factors (outgrowths of the interplay of muscular contractions coupled with the integrational mechanisms of the spinal cord) yields some unity or coherence to evolving movements, particularly in the case of gross bodily activities.

Eccles' dynamic loop hypothesis has been given empirical support by Evarts (1979), who implanted microelectrodes in the motor cortex of monkeys and observed significant differences in information-processing time during the early and late stages of acquisition. The initial phase of learning was characterized by a processing time of 200 msc. This time equals that required for the processing of kinesthetic feedback from peripheral receptors through the lower (spino-cerebellar) loop. When the animal developed proficiency in performing the task (manipulating a lever), information-processing time decreased to 40 msc. Evarts views this finding as substantiation of the existence of an upper loop linking the cerebellum to the cortex. This loop expedites the flow of information by enabling the cerebellum to employ data to regulate and control the evolving movement through feedforward.

Kornhuber (1974) theorizes that in the case of extremely rapid movements, such as the eye-hand coordinations characteristic of ball sports, the time required for regulation based upon feedback would simply be too great to allow for the successful execution of those skills. Kornhuber believes that the cerebellum is preprogramed to adjust a movement during the course of its execution. According to this view, the cerebellum becomes a master timeclock, regulating and controlling efferent discharge according to precoded temporal and spatial instructions.

What respective roles genetic coding and learning experience play in the programing of the cerebellar cortex remains equivocal. The classical view of the nervous system has it that only the cerebral cortex manifests a degree of plasticity sufficient for learning and the lower brain centers merely execute subroutines which have been genetically predetermined. The relative isolation of the structures comprising the cerebellar cortex lends credence to the argument that associative functions cannot be carried out to any significant degree at this level. Kornhuber argues that in the case of highly speeded movements, such as oculomotor responses, the concept of servoregulation through a dynamic loop cannot provide an adequate explanation due to the amount of time required for any loop system to function. As an alternative explanation, he proposes a chain-like arrangement in which afferent information relayed to the cerebellum from the preceding activity becomes a stimulus for eliciting the succeeding response in an encoded movement sequence. The extent to which the encoding of these sequences rests in genetic programing, as opposed to experiential factors, is not known.

Eccles, Ito, and Szentagothai (1967) speculate that there is a direct interaction between experiential factors and the structure and function of the cerebellum. He proposes that the cerebellum is not merely a fixed computing device, but a neuronal mechanism which is programable (capable of learning from experience) and which plays a major role in the execution of all skilled movement. He writes that the learning of skilled movement may be accompanied by actual structural changes (growth) of the secondary spines of Purkinje cell dendrites. It is theorized that the microgrowth of these structures results in increased synaptic function which consequently enables the cerebellum to compute in a specially adapted way for each movement. This information is stored and then recalled in order to provide the appropriate corrective action which keeps the movement on target.

### Peripheral Receptors

The integrative action of the motor sensory cortex and the cerebellum in the control of movement requires interoceptive and exteroceptive information from peripheral receptors. Receptors whose fibers give rise principally to conscious sensation are classified as exteroceptors; those whose output gives rise to regulatory adjustments effected below the level of consciousness are classified as interoceptors. All receptors, however, share certain properties regardless of the nature of their output.

The generator potentials elicited by the stimulation of nerve receptors are graded and vary in their frequency and amplitude, contrasted to the action potential, which is propagated along the nerve axon in an all-or-none fashion and varies only in its frequency. A distinct advantage of the generator potential is that a series of stimuli can build or summate and ultimately elicit an action potential, even though each individual stimulus impinging upon the receptor is itself of subthreshold intensity and, therefore, not powerful enough to excite the neuron. A receptor's capacity for generating graded potentials serves as a mechanism for screening out irrelevant input. Since there are millions of stimuli impinging upon an organism at any instant, the capacity to summate this input provides a mechanism for distinguishing critical sensory information from random environmental stimulation. The more critical the information, the more likely those stimuli will be repeated and the impulses summated to trigger a train of action potentials. Conversely, the more random the output, the less likely for it to be repeated and for its impulses to summate.

The afferent information processed by the motor sensory cortex and the cerebellum is generated by specialized receptors (proprioceptors) which respond to mechanical stimulation (stretch). Proprioceptors are located in the muscles and tendons, and constitute the sensory apparatus of the motor system. Specialized proprioceptors whose main function is conveying information about the position of the body are located in the neck region. Proprioceptors function as transducers by translating mechanical stimulation caused by changes in muscular force or limb displacement into nerve impulses which are relayed to kinesthetic association areas of the brain. There are essentially three types of kinesthetic feedback: information about the length of the muscle, the velocity of contraction, and the tension or force of contraction. Information about the length of the muscle and the velocity of contraction is conveyed by the muscle spindle. Information about the tension in the muscle is conveyed by the Golgi tendon organ.

*The Muscle Spindle.* The muscle spindle is one of the most important proprioceptors. Located in the contractile bundles of skeletal muscles and concentrated toward their centers, the number of spindles varies with the function of a given muscle.* The muscle spindle (comprised of intrafusal contractile fibers) lies in parallel to the extrafusal contractile fibers of the muscle itself and is unloaded, or silenced, by muscular contraction and excited by muscular stretch. The afferent discharge of a

---

*Granit (1970) writes that muscles that undergo only short variations in length are generally characterized by high levels of spindle control.

muscle spindle can be elicited in response to static as well as dynamic changes within the muscle.*

Since muscular stretch is one of the primary output variables in the control of movement, specialized receptors exist within the spindle for phasic and tonic muscular activity. Primary receptors (annulospirals) provide the spindle with position sensitivity (which conveys information about existing muscular length) and velocity sensitivity (which conveys information about changes in muscular length). Secondary receptors (flower sprays) have a relatively insignificant dynamic phase and are best adapted to signaling instantaneous length and length that has been maintained over time.

The muscle spindle is composed of two histologically distinct types of intrafusal fibers: the nuclear chain and the nuclear bag. According to Eyzaguirre and Fidone (1975), the "typical spindle" contains two nuclear bag fibers and four or five nuclear chain fibers. The annulospiral or primary receptor is formed by the larger afferent fibers (group Ia) coiling about the equatorial regions of the nuclear bag and the nuclear chain fibers. The flower spray or secondary receptor ending is formed by the smaller afferent fibers (group Ib) which terminate primarily upon the nuclear chain fibers.

In addition to its ability to react passively to stretch, the muscle spindle can be actively stimulated through its own motor fibers conveying information directly from the motor cortex. (The muscle spindle appears to be the only sensory receptor so endowed.) In the execution of complex movement, the efferent discharge of the motor cortex emanates from the activation of larger and smaller pyramidal neurons. Larger pyramidal neurons, or Betz cells, give rise to the skeletomotor or alpha fibers which innervate the muscle itself (the extrafusal fibers). Smaller pyramidal neurons give rise to fusimotor or gamma fibers which innervate the muscle spindle (the intrafusal fibers). (See Figure 6-9) The fusimotor fibers are themselves divisible into two groups: dynamic fibers, which increase the dynamic response of the primary spindle afferent but exert little or no effect upon spindle secondaries; and static fibers, which increase the static response of the primary and secondary spindle afferents.** The skeletomotor and

___

*Dynamic or phasic response is caused by a change in the length of a spindle. Static or tonic response results when the spindle is stretched to a constant length over a period of time.

**It is believed that static fibers terminate as trail endings upon the nuclear chain fibers and that dynamic fibers terminate as plate endings upon the nuclear bag fibers.

fusimotor fibers, along with the primary and secondary spindle afferents, collectively comprise one of the most important mechanisms in the control of movement, the gamma loop.

### Figure 6-9

### THE GAMMA LOOP

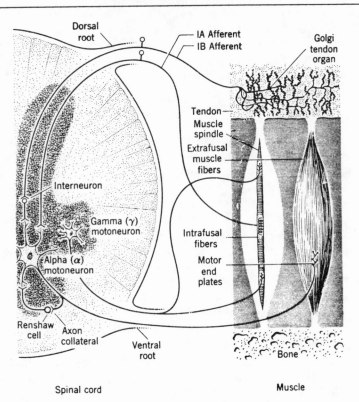

Spinal cord                                            Muscle

Although the structural differences between alpha and gamma fibers are well known, their respective functions in the control of movement are unclear. It was initially believed that the purpose of the gamma or fusimotor fibers was solely to exert a "follow-up" effect upon the muscle spindle. Since contraction of the extrafusal fibers would cause the spindle to slacken (thereby unloading or silencing it), it was held that fusimotor innervation readjusted the spindle to the changed length of the muscle. Once reset, the spindle could again communicate information on the state of the muscle. Further investigation of spindle function led to speculation that fusimotor (gamma) innervation actually preceded the alpha innervation of the muscle itself. This position was predicated upon the belief that presetting (biasing) the spindle would result in more precise motor regulation because the information conveyed to the spindle would be fed back to the skeletomotor neuron innervating the muscle. The spindle would then function as a template for refining the response of the motoneuron at that same segmental level of the spinal cord.

Current evidence (Smith, 1976), however, indicates that the intrafusal and extrafusal muscles are simultaneously innervated. This alpha-gamma coactivation provides a mechanism which can rapidly effect corrections in muscular force at the level of the spinal cord (through feedback loops between the spindle afferents and the skeletomotor neuron) as a movement is evolving. Since it is through the mechanism of alpha-gamma coactivation that the muscle and the spindle receive the same information at the same time, a system of checks and balances is established which ensures that the actual response will not depart significantly from the intended response. The coactivation mechanism is particularly effective in rapid compensation for unexpected changes (caused by such factors as muscular fatigue or air resistance). Since muscular adjustments can be effected in as little as 10 msc., this mechanism prevents an evolving movement pattern from being unduly affected by random environmental and physiological fluctuations.

The muscle spindle is the most important of the proprioceptors. It serves three major functions in the regulation and control of movement. The first entails servoregulatory activity. The length of the spindle must be continually adjusted to match that of the muscle. Because it lies in parallel to the muscle, muscular stretch will excite the spindle, increasing its afferent output. Conversely, muscular contraction causes the spindle to slacken and its output to cease. As the spindle is ineffective in the slackened state, compensatory adjustments must be effected in order to reset it to match the new length of the muscle. The servoregulatory function of the spindle enables it to adjust to changes in muscular length. Once its tension has been readjusted, the spindle is again capable of transmitting information concerning the state of the the muscle.

The second function is to provide proprioceptive information on the magnitude and velocity of muscular stretch. This information is relayed to higher centers in the nervous system where it is used in the direction and control of movement.

The third function pertains to the spindle's role in the reflexive regulation of coordinated movement and in the maintenance of posture. Stretching the spindle results in an afferent discharge which feeds back

upon the skeletomotor neuron (the homonymous motoneuron), innervating the muscle in which the spindle lies. The activation of the spindle
through stretch, therefore, results in facilitating skeletomotor neuron
discharge to the muscle itself, causing it to contract. (Stretching the
spindle results in the reflexive contraction of the homonymous muscle.)
In addition to stimulating its own muscle to contract, the spindle
inhibits skeletomotor discharge to the antagonistic muscle. This dual
phenomenon is known as reciprocal inhibition.

Since the muscles in the body are arranged antagonistically (for each
group of muscles exerting a movement in a given direction, there is an
opposing group which exerts its effect in an equal and opposite
direction), all forms of coordinated movement are dependent upon the
capacity to inhibit the function of the antagonistic muscle groups.
Reciprocal inhibition, in addition to its role in the coordination of
movement, is central in the reflexive control of posture. The maintenance
of posture is dependent upon sustained contraction of the antigravity
muscles. Any sudden stretching of these muscles (such as the knees
buckling from fatigue) is rapidly corrected through the myotatic stretch
reflex. This sudden stretching of the spindles in the antigravity muscles
results in the reflexive contraction of those muscles.

A common example of the myotatic stretch reflex is the knee jerk or
patellar reflex. Tapping the tendon results in a sudden stretch of the
spindle which causes the muscle to contract. The result is the rapid
extension of the knee. In order for this response to occur, however, all
the muscles antagonistic to the ongoing movement must be reciprocally
inhibited. It is the reflexive stimulation of the antigravity muscles
coupled with the reciprocal inhibition of their antagonists which enables
a person to maintain an upright posture without the need for cognitive
involvement.

*The Golgi Tendon Organ.* The muscle spindle is the most important
peripheral mechanism in motor control. Eccles (1973) writes that of all
the peripheral receptors, it is the information from the spindle which is
of greatest significance in the regulation of movement by higher centers.
The function of the spindle is augmented, however, by a second group
of muscle proprioceptors, the Golgi tendon organs (GTO). Each GTO
lies in series with the muscle and provides information concerning
muscle tension. Muscle contraction causes the spindle to slacken and to
relax or unload at the same time that it causes increased tension of the
muscle's tendons of insertion, thus exciting the GTO. Although the
GTO is located in series with the tendon and the muscle, a position
which enables it to respond equally to stretch and contraction, it is far

more sensitive to contractile force than to stretch. The reason for this behavior lies not in any inherent property of the GTO, but instead in the fact that much of the force generated during muscular stretch (particularly in the case of passive stretch) is absorbed by the elongation of the muscle cells. From a purely mechanical standpoint, more force is transferred to the GTO when the muscle contracts than when it stretches.

Considerable uncertainty existed about the role of the Golgi tendon organ in the control of movement. It was initially viewed merely as a safety mechanism with the purpose of preventing injury caused by over-contraction of the muscle. This view was reinforced by observations which revealed that the afferent (Ib) fibers emanating from the tendon organs of a given muscle exert a negative feedback effect upon the motoneuron innervating that muscle. (The contraction of the muscle stretches the tendon, exciting the GTO to transmit an afferent impulse which impinges upon the motoneuron, inhibiting it from further contraction of the muscle. [See Figure 6-10].) Current evidence has revealed that the GTO exerts an important function in the transmission of proprioceptive information in the monitoring and regulation of movement. Just as the spindle responds to static and dynamic stretch, the GTO responds to the velocity and duration of muscular tension. The spindle and the GTO function synergistically, i.e., those muscular conditions which tend to unload or silence the spindle excite the GTO.

_Articular Receptors._ The function of the muscle proprioceptors (the spindle and the GTO) is augmented by specialized receptors in the joints (articular receptors) which convey information pertaining to the position and the velocity of a given limb segment. Articular receptors are divided into three groups:

1. Transient detectors, which respond whenever the joint is moved, regardless of direction. Transient detectors respond to acceleration even when the joint is only vibrated.
2. Velocity detectors, which produce a continuous discharge which varies in its frequency in proportion to the rate of the movement. The faster the movement, the higher the frequency of the output; the slower the movement, the lower the discharge frequency.
3. Position-velocity detectors, which possess static and dynamic properties. These receptors are capable of conveying information concerning the position of a joint in the absence of movement and information concerning the velocity of a joint during movement.

Feedback from the articular receptors conveys information concerning the velocity and position of the joints of the body to central association

**Figure 6-10**

## GOLGI TENDON ORGAN
## COMPONENT OF THE LOCAL CONTROL SYSTEM

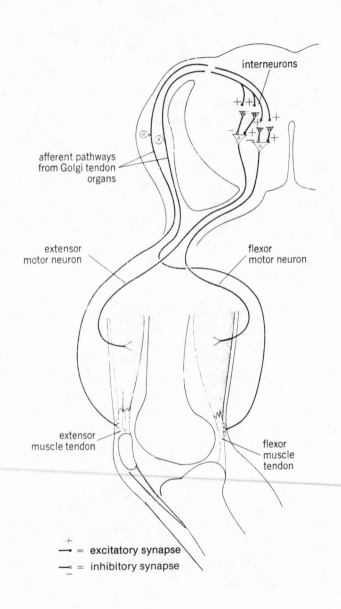

interneurons

afferent pathways
from Golgi tendon
organs

extensor
motor neuron

flexor
motor neuron

extensor
muscle tendon

flexor
muscle
tendon

$\overset{+}{\longrightarrow}$ = excitatory synapse

$\overset{}{\longrightarrow\!\circ}_{-}$ = inhibitory synapse

areas in the cortex. This information provides the learner with a knowledge of the relative position of the parts of his own body (position sense).

*Mechanoreceptors.* Proprioceptive input from the muscles and tendons is augmented by exteroceptive information which gives rise to the conscious awareness of limb position. This sensation is known as kinesthesia and is vital to a person's capacity to recognize body and limb position without the aid of visual and tactile information. The cutaneous mechanoreceptors are the most important exteroceptors in the regulation and control of movement and are sensitive to changes in position (static displacement), velocity (dynamic displacement), and direction. The directional sensitivity of these receptors is itself divisible into two sub-capacities: linear directionality and spatial directionality. The former relates to the discrimination of changes in position which are initiated from different starting points. If a movement consists of flexing the elbow to a position of 90°, the discharge pattern of the directional receptors would vary depending upon the initial position of the joint. (A different pattern results if the movement is initiated from a position of 30° flexion rather than from one of 60° flexion.) Spatial directionality pertains to the property of certain receptors to respond only to movements in a particular direction, such as those proceeding from left to right or from a position of flexion to one of extension.

### The Spinal Cord

In order for the information generated by the peripheral receptors to be utilized in motor control, it must first be integrated and then relayed to higher centers within the nervous system for further processing. The integrating mechanisms inherent in the structure of the spinal cord embody the first phase in the central processing of peripheral input. A cross-sectional view of the spinal cord reveals two major structural divisions: a central "H"-shaped body composed of gray matter, and a surrounding area of white matter which comprises the outer area of the cord. The gray matter is itself divisible into two major structural segments: the anterior and posterior gray horns. These horns divide the white matter into four areas or funiculi: a dorsal or posterior funiculus, a ventral or anterior funiculus, and two lateral funiculi. (See Figure 6-11)

The white matter consists of myelinated nerve fibers which comprise the ascending and descending pathways of the spinal cord. These pathways or tracts either 1) connect different segments of the spinal cord (intersegmental pathways, which either ascend or descend but

**Figure 6-11**

## CROSS-SECTION OF SPINAL CORD

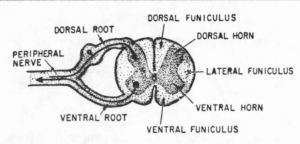

remain within the cord); 2) convey either proprioceptive or exteroceptive afferent information to higher centers in the brain (ascending pathways); or 3) convey efferent output from these higher centers to motoneurons (descending pathways).

The gray matter contains the cell bodies of motoneurons, collateral fibers of afferent neurons, and interneuronal pools which integrate sensory and motor information. The cell bodies of alpha motoneurons (which innervate extrafusal muscle through skeletomotor fibers) and gamma motoneurons (which innervate intrafusal muscle through fusimotor fibers) are located in the ventral horn of the gray matter. The cell bodies of afferent neurons, in contrast, lie outside the spinal cord in the dorsal root ganglion. (See Figure 6-12) The postganglionic fibers of afferent neurons, upon entering the cord, show marked divergence, giving rise to branches or collaterals. These collaterals either ascend or descend through the white matter, or else they directly penetrate the dorsal gray horn at the same segmental level at which they enter.

Afferent collaterals which penetrate the gray horn at the same segment at which they enter the cord can either synapse directly with skeletomotor neurons or enter an interneuronal pool. The only known example of the former phenomenon in humans is the myotatic stretch reflex, in which the primary afferent from a muscle projects directly (monosynaptically) to the homonymous skeletomotor neuron (the motorneuron innervating the same muscle in which the spindle lies). Afferent collaterals which enter interneuronal pools make diffuse (polysynaptic) connections before terminating upon their target motoneurons. Afferent collaterals which form monosynaptic connections terminate only upon skeletomotor neurons; those which form polysynaptic connections may terminate upon either skeletomotor or fusimotor neurons.

Afferent collaterals which make polysynaptic connections upon

## Figure 6-12

## SPINAL CORD ORGANIZATION

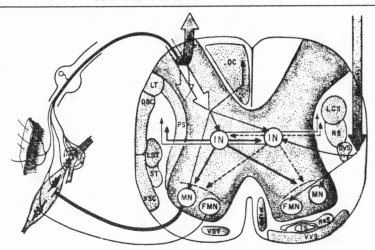

Schematic representation of spinal cord organization, showing neuronal routes to segmental, ascending and descending pathways. (For explanation see text.) Segmental elements: *IN*, interneuron pools; *MN*, motoneuron pools (skeletomotor neurons, or ∝ motoneurons); *FMN*, fusimotor neurons (Υ motoneurons). Ascending sensory pathways (shown on left half of spinal cord): *DC*, dorsal columns; *PS*, propriospinal system; *LT*, Lissauer's tract; *LST*, lateral spinothalamic tract; *VST*, ventral spinothalamic tract; *ST*, spinotectal tract. Descending motor pathways (shown on right half of spinal cord): *LCS*, lateral corticospinal tract; *VCS*, ventral corticospinal tract; *RS*, rubrospinal tract; *DVS*, dorsal vestibulospinal tract; *VVS*, ventral vestibulospinal tract; *ReS*, reticulospinal tract; *TS*, tectospinal tract.

penetrating the gray horn terminate in interneuronal pools which lie either on the same (ipsilateral) side of the cord as their point of entry or on the opposite (contralateral) side. There are several interneuronal pools at each segment of the spinal cord, located between the dorsal and ventral gray horns. Interneuronal pools on both sides of the spinal cord are in communication with one another, and each pool makes synaptic connections with skeletomotor and fusimotor neurons lying on the ipsilateral and contralateral sides of the cord. The transfer of information from dorsal to ventral roots within the cord is extremely complex and is characterized by high degrees of divergence and convergence. Upon entering the dorsal root, afferent fibers diverge, giving rise to a large number of collaterals. In the ventral root, a single skeletomotor neuron can receive information converging from as many as 5,000 synaptic inputs. It is through the divergence and convergence of afferent input that efferent output is ultimately refined and focused. The net result of these complex neuronal interactions is sensory motor integration at the segmental level of the spinal cord.

The intersegmental circuitry of the cord constitutes a preprogramed mechanism which functions in the control of fundamental stereotyped responses (e.g., the simple reflex). These responses are effected with great speed, but are highly circumscribed by the information-processing capacity of the segmental neuronal circuits. The intraspinal regulation of more complex motor responses, therefore, depends upon the transfer of information through intersegmental pathways, such as the propriospinal system. The fibers of the propriospinal tract (afferent collaterals and interneurons) remain intraspinal and link different levels of the cord. These fibers ascend or descend for several segments from their point of origin and then reenter the gray horn to synapse with interneurons or motoneurons at that level. Intersegmental intraspinal pathways play a key role in the reflexive coordination of the movements of the upper and lower extremities, such as those employed in walking and running.

Although intraspinal mechanisms are central to the regulation of complex reflex activities, the initiation and control of purposive, goal-directed movements is dependent upon the intervention of higher centers in the nervous system. These centers continually modify their output in response to information feedback conveyed through ascending pathways from receptors in the periphery. Proprioceptive information from the muscle spindle and the tendon organ is conveyed to the cerebellum through the spino-cerebellar and spino-olivary tracts; extero-ceptive information from cutaneous and articular receptors is conveyed through the dorsal column pathway. Fibers in the dorsal column pathway project to the cerebral cortex; proprioceptive pathways terminate at the level of the cerebellum. The spino-cerebellar tract terminates as mossy fibers, and the spino-olivary tract gives rise to the climbing fibers.

While most of the individual fibers which comprise the proprioceptive tracts tend to relay information from the spindles and tendon organs of restricted groups of muscles, there are certain fibers which convey information from single muscles or groups of synergistic muscles. The firing pattern of a given tract tends to resemble that of the receptor it serves. Those fibers which convey information from muscle spindle receptors will show increased activity during muscular stretch and decreased activity during muscular contraction. Conversely, fibers which convey information from the tendon organ receptors manifest increased activity during muscular contraction and decreased activity during stretch.

Eyzaguirre and Fidone (1975) write that all pathways ascending from the spinal cord to the cerebellum share a number of common features, regardless of the specific nature of the information they convey (e.g., input from muscle, skin, or joint). All ascending pathways terminate in the cerebellar hemisphere ipsilateral to the point at which they enter the cord. Afferent collaterals which penetrate the right side of the spinal cord will terminate in the right cerebellar hemisphere, and those which enter on the left side will terminate in the left cerebellar hemisphere. In addition to their pattern of communicating information ipsilaterally, these ascending pathways are all designed to reproduce the peripheral sensory message quickly and accurately. Conduction time in these pathways ranges between 40 and 110 msc., and there are a minimal number of synapses. In fact, with the exception of the spino-olivary tract which makes three synaptic connections, all ascending tracts to the cerebellum have only two synaptic connections between the peripheral afferent fibers and their target neurons.

The dorsal column pathway conveys exteroceptive information directly to the cerebral cortex, making only three synaptic connections along the way. The primary afferent fibers from the cutaneous and articular peripheral receptors synapse with second order neurons in the medulla. These neurons ascend to the ventrobasal complex in the thalamus, where they synapse with third order neurons which project directly to the sensory motor cortex. Sensory input is translated into conscious experience through the specialized nuclei found in each of the three levels. These nuclei possess the capacity to reproduce accurately the sensory messages generated by the various types of peripheral sensory receptors.

The processing of exteroceptive information entails the convergence of many peripheral inputs into a common ascending pathway which itself diverges at different levels of the brain. The accurate localization of peripheral stimuli is ensured, however, through two neuronal mechanisms which act to focus nuclear cells on a given input. These mechanisms are wired into the synaptic circuitry of the dorsal column nuclei in the medulla and are designed to restore the acuity of peripheral discrimination by offsetting the effects of convergence and divergence. In effect, they function as decoders which unscramble the encoded neural message and reproduce it in its original form. The neurological processes which underlie this sensory decoding are known collectively as lateral inhibition. This phenomenon is essential to the processing of exteroceptive input by higher centers. Its effects are manifested in such complex behavioral activities as habituation and selective attention. The athlete's ability to screen out both the noise of the spectators and the spurious movements of opposing players, simultaneously devoting full attention to the critical aspects of the game situation, is a prime example of the behavioral effects of lateral inhibition.

Although input from proprioceptors in muscles and tendons is not conveyed to the sensory motor cortex through a direct pathway and does not give rise to conscious sensation, Eccles (1973) contends that this proprioceptive information is nonetheless central to the regulation and control of volitional movement. He writes that information from the primary spindle afferent is conveyed to the cortex through a complex network of synaptic relays and that its major purpose is to provide continuous feedback concerning the length of the muscles involved in the ongoing movement. This information does not, however, give rise to an immediate conscious awareness of the evolving movement. Instead, it provides the learner with a subtle, almost subconscious perception of it. This proprioceptive feedback provides information which is critical in motor learning. It is a frame of reference which enables the learner to assess the degree of discrepancy between the motor commands effected by the cerebral cortex and the actual response of the muscles. This discrepancy between the movement desired and the one that actually occurs enables the learner to formulate an image or proprioceptive illusion of a given motor act. The greater the mismatch between the desired response and the one attained, the more vivid the illusion. Conversely, when there is little or no mismatch, the illusion is minimal. The more effectively the cortical commands are executed, the less the learner is aware of proprioceptive feedback.

Roland (1978) writes that the conscious perception of movement is dependent upon information-processing functions which entail feedback and feedforward mechanisms. Predicated upon experimental observation, Roland's argument is that information feedback generated by the proprioceptors in the muscles and tendons is ultimately relayed to the level of the cerebral cortex, where it is employed in modifying the motor command governing the ongoing movement. The feedforward information relayed to the cortical association areas consists of a copy of the motor command to the involved muscle groups. This efference copy or corollary discharge is believed to convey information about such movement parameters as position, magnitude, force, and estimated load. The feedforward aspect of motor control gives rise to the conscious awareness of movement and serves as a template or reference mechanism for processing feedback from the peripheral receptors. Roland confirms Eccles' contention that the conscious awareness of movement is due to the degree of the perceived mismatch between the response desired and the one attained.

The descending pathways are the final link in the communication network which integrates central and peripheral neurological processes. With the exception of the cortico-spinal tracts arising from the cerebral cortex, all descending tracts originate from the brain stem. The plasticity and adaptability of motor behavior is largely a result of the action of these descending pathways, which modify the stereotyped response patterns programed into the segmental circuits of the spinal cord. The descending tracts are aimed primarily toward two distinct segmental targets: the interneuronal pools and the individual skeleto-motor and fusimotor neurons. Although the information conveyed by the interneuronal pools is ultimately relayed to the skeletomotor and fusimotor neurons, it is the degree of direct projection to the motoneurons which is indicative of the capacity for skilled movement. The higher this degree of direct projection, the greater the precision and finesse with which a movement can be effected.

*Environmental and Neurological Interactions*

The execution of complex, goal-directed patterns of movement is dependent upon the interaction between centers in the cerebral cortex which mediate conscious experience and those in the spinal cord which serve in the stereotyped regulation of reflexive responses. Cognition and insight into the nature of a complex motor skill are necessary during the initial phase of its acquisition. It is exceedingly difficult to learn a task in the absence of knowledge of its purpose and the manner in which it is to be executed. As proficiency is developed, however, the cognitive information employed in the initial acquisition of the task becomes internalized and serves as a reference mechanism or template in the regulation of specific behaviors.

An athlete in a game situation does not have time to verbalize and to reason; responses are based upon ability to process exteroceptive and proprioceptive information quickly and accurately. This information concerns the actual temporal and spatial characteristics of the ongoing activity, such as the position and speed of the involved limb segments in relation to the ball or other object of play and the whereabouts of supporting and opposing players. Although nonverbal in its nature, this information is processed in a systematic manner in response to instructions laid down by cognitive structures (memory stores) which are themselves programed with information concerning the rules and principles governing a given activity.

Although motor learning entails the integration of higher-order neural processes with fundamental reflexive activities in the processing of environmental input, the questions concerning the actual interactions between experience and neurological functioning remain largely unanswered. The extent to which the ability to acquire motor skills is predetermined by the structural and functional limitations of the nervous system is not yet understood. There are arguments espousing the extreme deterministic position which holds that the level of proficiency an individual can attain is largely predetermined by hereditary factors. On the other end of the spectrum, there are those who argue that in the absence of any pathological impairments, experience and motivation rather than hereditary factors are the critical elements in learning. Current research has shown that neither of these extreme positions is completely adequate as there tends to be an interaction between factors in the environment and the functioning of the nervous system. Even though the neurological circuitry is intact, environmental stimulation appears critical to its optimal functioning.

Eccles (1973) theorizes that the physical basis of learning lies in the plasticity of the synapse because strong activation will result in the growth of synaptic microstructures, lack of stimulation will result in their atrophy. He cites experimental evidence which revealed that repeated stimulation of skeletomotor neurons resulted in a sixfold increase in the magnitude of their post-synaptic excitatory potentials. The extent of such synaptic modification appears to vary with different types of neurons. No synaptic potentiation was observed when primary spindle afferents were repeatedly stimulated.

In order to link modifications in the microstructure of a synapse to learning, it is necessary to demonstrate that phenomena such as synaptic potentiation are lasting and that they will persist for prolonged periods of time following the cessation of stimulation. Eccles reports that although post-synaptic potentiation in spinal neurons was almost doubled following rapid stimulation, all traces of potentiation disappeared within a few minutes following the cessation of stimulation. These findings were not unexpected, however, since neither learning nor memory is believed to be a function of the spinal cord. In contrast, stimulation of neurons in the hippocampus, an area of the cerebral cortex believed to be important in memory, resulted in synaptic potentiation for periods as long as ten hours following the cessation of excitation.

Eccles cites experimental evidence which indicates that these modifiable synapses are most prominent in the higher levels of the brain, and adds that they may well be the physical basis of learning and memory. The contention that these synapses are central in the mediation of complex behavioral activities is substantiated, at least in part, by evidence which indicates that they regress through disuse. Eccles argues, however, that use and disuse do not, in and of themselves, constitute wholly satisfactory explanations of the neurological phenomena associated with complex behavioral activity. In the absence of pathological impairment, all synapses in the brain are active, and there must be some special mechanism, other than use alone, which underlies synaptic modification. The conjunction theory of learning is a viable attempt at resolving this issue. The theory postulates the existence of specialized synapses which provide instructions for the growth and modification of surrounding activated synapses. Such modification is believed to depend upon the synthesis of specific proteins which provide the physical basis for the synaptic microgrowth which is thought to underlie learning and memory.

Granit (1977) theorizes that the physical basis of learning entails the establishment of specific synaptic connections within the central nervous system. Neurons whose axons project over long distances (e.g., those which give rise to ascending or descending fibers or to skeletomotor or fusimotor fibers) make synaptic connections which are wholly predetermined by specific biological (genetic) programing. In contrast, the synaptic connections of neurons which give rise to axons traversing only short distances (e.g., interneurons) are believed to result from the interaction between flexible, open-ended genetic programing and specific environmental stimulation. The former type of synaptic connections is most commonly found in the peripheral pathways which link muscles and muscle proprioceptors with the central nervous system; the latter type is most prevalent within the central nervous system, particularly within the cerebral cortex. Open synapses are believed to account for the plasticity which characterizes cortical development during infancy and early childhood.

Although the cortical plasticity resulting from the interaction of environmental stimulation and biological programing is believed to terminate by early adolescence, an individual is nonetheless capable of learning throughout his life. Granit theorizes that in the mature individual, the capacity of the nervous system to adapt to changing environmental conditions may be a function of specialized synapses which are ordinarily inactive and held in reserve until they are called upon to meet the demands of a novel learning situation. He cites experimental evidence indicating that certain synapses which projected upon muscles and appeared normal in all respects were actually found to be inactive during motor activity which involved those muscles. He contends that these findings may indicate that neural adaptability in the mature organism is a function of the activation and deactivation of existing synaptic pathways rather than a result of the formation of new ones.

These current findings which reveal the interaction between environmental stimulation and the structure and function of the nervous system have given rise to a changing view of the role of neurological processes in the mediation of complex behavioral activities. Until the middle of this century, problems associated with learning and teaching were viewed primarily within the context of behavioristic theory. Learning was mistakenly regarded as a passive process in which the responses of the learner, both verbal and motor, could be manipulated through the use of various schedules of reinforcement. However, advances in knowledge of the interrelationships between the structure of the brain and behavior (particularly in the case of the major and minor cortical hemispheres) coupled with a greater understanding of information-processing mechanisms (derived from advances in computer technology) have drastically altered the long-standing theoretical views of learning. Learning is currently regarded as an active dynamic process in which there is continual interaction between the learner and the environment.

Since the acquisition of complex, goal-directed motor skills entails the coordinated interaction of central and peripheral neurological processes, the teaching of these skills must account for individual differences in the information-processing capacities of the learner. Bogen (1977) writes that the hemispheric specialization of the cerebral cortex provides the learner with the capacity for processing two distinctly different modes of sensory input. The major or dominant hemisphere is central in the performance of conceptual activities, which entail orderly logical operations. This hemisphere processes verbal information that is written or spoken. The minor or nondominant hemisphere, in contrast, is critical in the performance of concrete practical activities, which pertain to prevailing environmental conditions. This hemisphere processes information that is visual or kinesthetic. (It also responds to sounds which are not verbal.) Bogen contends that given this hemispheric specialization, learning will be best facilitated by teaching methods which employ verbal as well as visual information. It is essential that verbal explanations be accompanied by visual demonstrations in the teaching of motor skills.

Although the teaching of motor skills should employ methods suited to the capacities of both cortical hemispheres, individuals differ in terms of the sensory modality to which they best respond. Contemporary society, as evidenced by the focus of formal education, tends to place greater value on skills related to capacities of the major hemisphere. Success in traditional academic areas is deemed more desirable than proficiency in creative activities or motor learning. Since individuals differ in their capacities for processing special types of sensory input,

Bogen suggests that educational priorities be reexamined. The educative process should not seek to force all individuals into a common mold but should strive to provide equal opportunity for success in verbal as well as motor activities. In order to achieve these ends, teaching methods and the aptitudes of the learner must be matched.

*References*

Barnes, C.D. and C. Kircher. *Readings in Neurophysiology.* New York: John Wiley, 1968.

Bogen, J.E. "Some Educational Implications of Hemispheric Specialization." *In* M.C. Wittrock et al. (eds.), *The Human Brain.* Englewood Cliffs, NJ: Prentice-Hall, 1977.

Brooks, V.B. "Information Processing in the Motorsensory Cortex." *In* K.N. Leibovic (ed.), *Information Processing in the Nervous System.* New York: Springer-Verlag, 1969.

Eccles, J.C. "The Dynamic Loop Hypothesis of Movement Control." *In* K.N. Leibovic (ed.), *Information Processing in the Nervous System.* New York: Springer-Verlag, 1969.

_____. *The Understanding of the Brain.* New York: McGraw-Hill, 1973.

_____. "Evolution of the Brain in Relation to the Development of the Self-Conscious Mind." *In* S.J. Dimond and D.A. Blizard (eds.), *Evolution and Lateralization of the Brain.* New York: The New York Academy of Sciences, 1977.

_____, M. Ito, and J. Szentagothai. *The Cerebellum as a Neuronal Machine.* New York: Springer-Verlag, 1967.

Evarts, E.V. "Representation of Movements and Muscles by Pyramidal Tract Neurons of the Precentral Motor Cortex." *In* M.D. Yahr and D.P. Purpura (eds.), *Neurophysiological Basis of Normal and Abnormal Motor Activities.* New York: Raven Press, 1967.

_____. "Brain Mechanisms of Movement." *Scientific American, 241 (3)* (1979), 164–179.

Eyzaguirre, C. and S.J. Fidone. *Physiology of the Nervous System.* 2nd ed. Chicago: Yearbook Medical Publishers, 1975.

Gawronski, R. *Bionics.* New York and Amsterdam: Elsevier, 1971.

Glencross, D.J. and M.M. Koreman. "The Processing of Proprioceptive Signals." *Neurophysiologia, 17* (1979), 683 – 687.

Granit, R. *The Basis of Motor Control.* New York: Academic Press, 1970.

_____. *The Purposive Brain.* Cambridge, Mass.: MIT Press, 1977.

Kaufman, A.S., R. Zalma, and N. L. Kaufman. "The Relationship of Hand Dominance to the Motor Coordination, Mental Ability and

Right-Left Awareness of Young Normal Children." *Child Development, 45* (1978), 885 – 888.

Kornhuber, H.H. "Cerebral Cortex, Cerebellum and Basal Ganglia: An Introduction to Their Motor Functions." *In* F.O. Schmitt and F.G. Worden (eds.), *The Neurosciences.* Cambridge, Mass.: MIT Press, 1974.

Luria, A.R. *Human Brain and Psychological Processes.* New York: Harper and Row, 1966.

Maiorov, V.I., E.I. Savchenko, and B.I. Kotlyar. "Transformation of the Afferent Tactile Signal Into a Motor Command in the Cat Motor Cortex." *Neuroscience and Behavioral Physiology, 10* (1980), 374–381.

McGlone, J. "Sex Differences in Human Brain Asymmetry: A Critical Survey." *The Behavioral and Brain Sciences, 3* (1980), 215–263.

Roland, P.E. "Sensory Feedback to the Cerebral Cortex During Voluntary Movement in Man." *The Behavioral and Brain Sciences, 1* (1978), 129–171.

Sherrington, C. *The Integrative Action of the Nervous System.* New Haven, Conn.: Yale University Press, 1948.

Smith, J.L. "Fusimotor Loop Properties and Involvement During Voluntary Movement." *In* J. Keogh and R.S. Hutton (eds.), *Exercise and Sport Sciences Reviews.* Santa Barbara, Cal.: Journal Publishing Affiliates, 1976.

Turkewitz, G. "The Development of Lateral Differentiation in the Human Infant." In S.J. Dimond and D.A. Blizard (eds.), *Evolution and Lateralization of the Brain.* New York: The New York Academy of Sciences, 1977.

Vander, A.J., J.H. Sherman, and D.S. Luciano. *Human Physiology: The Mechanisms of Body Function.* 2nd ed. New York: McGraw-Hill, 1975.

# CHAPTER 7

# Ability Factors in Motor Learning

THE NERVOUS SYSTEM is the integrative mechanism in the dynamic interaction between the learner and the environment. Qualitative distinctions in the learner's capacity to adapt to a given situation are manifested as individual differences within a class of behavioral traits known as ability factors. There is considerable theoretical speculation about the degree to which such factors result from specific experience or innate biological programing. There is also controversy about the extent to which they serve in predetermining the rate and the upper limit of learning.

The study of ability factors in motor learning is marked by a number of controversies: the appropriate methodological techniques for the identification and assessment of motor abilities; the role of ability factors in the learning and performance of motor skills; the very existence of ability factors themselves. The extreme views concerning the role of ability factors in learning are reflected in the opposing theoretical positions of the behaviorists and the biological determinists.

Behaviorism (as espoused by Watson) is predicated upon the position that learning and proficiency are solely the result of experiential and environmental factors. An individual manifests a propensity for acquiring a given activity not because of the presence of inherent ability factors but because of exposure to environmental situations which strengthen particular response patterns. According to the behavioristic position, cultural factors bear most heavily upon an individual's capacity to acquire particular skills and far outweigh the effects of any organismic or biological factors. Individuals from upper-level socio-economic backgrounds, for example, are exposed to situations which stress the development of verbal skills, such as parental attention in the form of reading. An individual from the lower socioeconomic classes is often forced to spend much of his time outside the home in the presence of his peers. In such environmental conditions motor activity tends to predominate heavily over verbal activity.

In contrast to the behavioristic position, biological determinists contend that ability is "wired in" at birth as the direct result of genetic programing. Advocates of determinism argue that experience will only magnify these innate differences because the progress of persons with high ability levels will be accelerated while that of the low-ability individual will increasingly lag behind. Biological determinists view abilities as factors which set severe limitations upon an individual's achievements in given areas of endeavor. Low ability levels are believed virtually to preclude the attainment of even a minimal degree of proficiency in an activity which is dependent upon those abilities. A person with low quantitative ability, for example, would be regarded as having a minimal chance of success in an algebra class, regardless of the time and effort he was willing to expend.

A position which attempts to reconcile these theoretical differences is espoused by the interactionists, who view ability as a function of environment and biology. Interactionists acknowledge the importance of biological programing in the development of abilities but argue that experiential factors (environmental stimulation) are a vital element in their shaping and refinement. Although a child may possess a level of neurological maturation which is sufficient to enable him or her to read, environmental stimulation must also be present in the actual development of reading ability. Interactionists see ability factors exhibiting a high degree of plasticity during youth and adolescence when they are greatly affected by learning and experience. In adulthood, however, these factors are believed to solidify and to represent more or less permanent behavioral traits which delineate particular capacities for processing given types of information (e.g., quantitative and verbal abilities).

Although determinists and interactionists both regard abilities as limiting factors in learning, the former view low ability as an insurmountable stumbling block in the path of learning. The latter argue that low ability does not preclude an individual's attaining a reasonable degree of success in a given activity, provided he is willing to expend a greater amount of effort to attain a given level of proficiency. However, the ultimate attainable degree of proficiency will most likely be lower for an individual with limited ability.

Noble (1978) writes that the role of heredity in human ability factors is not yet clearly understood. However, it is reasonable to assume that genetic endowment along with environmental opportunity and experience plays a functional role in the development of these factors and in the levels of proficiency ultimately attained. This contention is substantiated by empirical evidence derived from the study of rhythmical ability. Forty-three percent of the variance of this ability was attributable to heredity, 57 percent to environmental factors. This ability is a significant factor in the acquisition of specific musical skills. Discrimination of rhythm is significantly correlated with rhythmic performance.

Those who can distinguish two rhythmical patterns, given the appropriate training, are more likely to produce those patterns than individuals who are given the same training but cannot discriminate.

McCauley et al. (1980) write that there is controversy concerning the role of environmental and biological factors in time perception. Determinists contend that this ability is a function of an internal biological clock which is genetically programed; behaviorists argue that it is merely a capacity for processing a specific type of information which develops through experience. The authors write that biological and experiential factors are both involved in the ability to perceive time, and that the respective importance of each varies with the specific nature of the criterion task. The perception of very brief time periods on the order of milliseconds is believed to be a function of innate biological mechanisms; perception of intervals on the order of several seconds is attributed to cognitive processes which are the product of learning and experience.

Controversy also exists concerning the distinctions between the concepts of abilities and of individual differences. Bechtoldt (1970) contends that the term "ability" is primarily confined to the description of behavioral traits and the term "individual differences" has a somewhat broader interpretation encompassing physiological and organismic variables as well. Motor learning theorists regard abilities as behavioral traits which accompany the individual in every learning situation and which account for differences in the rate of acquisition and the ultimate level of proficiency attained.

### Defined and Inferred Ability Factors

Bechtoldt further writes that there are two ways in which an ability can be empirically described: 1) in terms of an actual value or score based upon performance on a single test (a defined ability); 2) in terms of a hypothetical value which is inferred through a complex statistical technique known as factor analysis (an inferred ability). Factor analysis entails the correlation of performance upon several different measures. Since an ability may be defined as a capacity to perform an act, it is often assessed in terms of a score on a single test which is specifically designed to measure that capacity. An individual's performance as measured by a dynamometer, for example, is often utilized as a direct measure or defined ability of strength. However, when no single test can satisfactorily measure an ability, it must be inferred in the form of a hypothetical value which is empirically derived through the correlational analysis of performance upon several tests (factor analysis). When performance upon a number of different skills appears to be related (e.g., pull-ups, chins, floor push-ups, and parallel bar push-ups or dips), the objective is to hypothesize the single factor or ability which underlies proficiency upon each of the individual skills in question. The underlying ability construct in the preceding example is hypothesized to be dynamic strength (muscular endurance).

According to Bechtoldt, defined measures of individual differences (test scores) may be used to represent either dependent or independent variables. In the former, there is little controversy concerning the assumption that observed interindividual differences in performance are valid representations of the degree of variability in the subjects' capacity to perform the criterion measure. It is reasonable to assume, for example, that in the majority of cases, subjects who perform well upon a test of a given skill possess a greater knowledge of the skill than do subjects who perform poorly—those with greater proficiency perform better than those without. There is, however, considerable disagreement over the latter (independent variables), particularly when they are employed as predictive indices which purport to measure pretask ability level. Since defined ability factors are predicated upon actual test scores, it may be rightfully argued that these scores reflect variations in the experience of the subject and the conditions under which the test was administered, as well as in actual ability level. Bechtoldt contends, however, that despite these limitations, defined ability measures can enjoy successful application to motor learning research, provided their use is confined to the prediction of behavior rather than to its explanation.

The utilization of inferred ability factors in behavioral research is far more complicated. Although inferred ability factors are hypothetical in nature, they must nonetheless be defined operationally if they are to be applied in behavioral research. In order to define explicitly a hypothetical variable, a single value must be derived which is based upon a composite of scores attained from performance upon several different tests. This procedure, unfortunately, is often unreliable since different researchers may inadvertently refer to the same factor by different names or use the same name to describe different factors.

In addition to the problems associated with the naming of ability factors, their identification is confounded by differences in the nature of the criterion tasks employed to measure these abilities, variations in the conditions under which these tasks were administered, differences in the subjects' experience with the criterion measures, and variations in the level of proficiency upon the criterion task demanded. Unless ability factors are derived under identical conditions and reflect identical behavioral traits, they are of little value in the study of behavior.

Bechtoldt concludes that defined ability factors may be freely employed as dependent as well as independent variables, as long as appropriate constraints are adopted in the latter case. Extreme caution must be employed in applying inferred ability constructs, however, in order to ensure that the conditions under which these factors have been derived are uniform and that each factor truly represents a single identifiable behavioral trait.

The use of defined ability factors in motor learning research was initiated by Brace (1926) and McCloy (1934) for the purpose of developing predictive indices concerned with assessing an individual's overall propensity for acquiring motor skills. Unfortunately, these measures employed skills which were highly specific in nature and therefore yielded findings greatly limited in scope. Current research concerning the role of ability factors in motor learning is predicated upon the derivation of hypothetical or inferred ability factors. These factors, once derived, are then employed to predict specific aspects of motor behavior rather than serving as predictive indices for the acquisition of all types of motor skills.

Since experimental research in motor learning is often based upon the assumption that individual differences in the abilities and capacities of the subjects merely constitute a source of error variance which will be randomized throughout the experimental groups (provided the appropriate sampling techniques have been employed), the concept of a behavioral baseline in the acquisition of motor skills is often ignored. Although motor skills are highly specific in nature, a proportion of the variance of every motor skill is concomitant with such factors as speed, endurance, flexibility, and strength relating to the initial state of the learner. In effect, precise prediction and control of motor behavior require stable baseline measures of an individual's abilities prior to experimental manipulation. There have been numerous attempts to develop instruments for assessing such baseline factors, but none have proven truly successful. Studies concerned with correlating performance upon tests of initial ability with performance upon specific motor skills have yielded conflicting results.

Research on the place of basic ability factors in motor learning has been characterized by a series of theoretical controversies. The primary issues have centered on the specificity versus the generality of these abilities and the respective roles played by nature and nurture in their development. Students of individual differences in motor learning are also divided over the relative stability or plasticity of motor ability factors. There is also marked disagreement over the nature of the interaction between these ability factors with the learning process itself.

Two important elements, further limiting the accuracy of the prediction of motor performance from pretrial measurements of ability, pertain to the limitations inherent in any procedure and to specific factors related to task taxonomy. Finally, the question, are individual differences in motor learning the result of behavioral traits which reflect the internal organization of the individual or merely artifacts of the taxonomy of a particular learning task, remains largely unanswered.

### Generality Versus Specificity

Early attempts at assessing the role of individual differences in motor learning were predicated upon a belief in the existence of a general motor ability factor which purportedly accounted for an individual's level of proficiency in the acquisition and the performance of all types of motor skills. Laboring under this assumption, Brace (1926) developed a motor ability test battery of thirty stunt-type items for the purpose of assessing the facility for the acquisition of new skills as well as the probable ultimate attainable level of proficiency following initial acquisition.

McCloy (1934) was also committed to the concept of a general motor ability factor. He argued the need to develop measures of motor aptitude which would be analogous to tests employed in assessing intelligence and would use items essentially unfamiliar to the subjects and relatively immune to the incremental effects of practice. Based upon this belief, McCloy (1937) modified the Brace Battery (the Iowa Revision) to include only twenty items, removing the tests which he felt reflected prior experience and practice rather than initial ability.

A third attempt to assess a general motor ability factor in learning may be seen in the work of Johnson (1932), who developed a ten-item stunt-type test for the purpose of assessing motor educability or the capacity for the acquisition of motor skills. Metheny (1938) reduced the Johnson test to four items only, observing that her shortened version correlated very highly (r =.98)  with the original longer form of the test.

The entire concept of general motor ability came under severe scrutiny, however, when the use of these tests as predictors of success in motor learning yielded highly inconsistent results. Although Metheny found that her revised version of the Johnson test correlated well with the acquisition of tumbling skills, Gire and Espenschade (1942) found that neither the original Johnson test, the Brace test, nor McCloy's Iowa Revision of the Brace test correlated well with performance upon team-sport skills.

These findings prompted Brace (1946) to reevaluate his position regarding general motor ability. He deduced that at least two types of motor ability must exist: one pertaining to the utilization of strength, speed, power, and dexterity in manipulating an external object, such as a ball; and a second which relates to the manipulation and control of the body itself without regard to an external object. Brace referred to the first as athletic ability and to the second as stunt-type ability. He argued that performance tests composed of items measuring the latter abilities are not valid predictors of success for the acquisition of sport skills and, conversely, that tests measuring athletic abilities are unrelated to performance upon stunt-type activities. He conceded the probability of the existence of many specific motor abilities and acknowledged that the fundamental concept of a general motor capacity factor was questionable.

McCraw (1949), through the application of factor analytic techniques, corroborated Brace's revised view that separate abilities exist for sport skills and stunt-type activities. McCraw identified three ability factors related to sport skills: dynamic object control without an implement; dynamic object control with an implement; and aiming control in static body position, as well as a single factor of body coordination related to the acquisition of stunt-type activities. Perhaps McCraw's most salient contribution to the understanding of the role of basic abilities in motor learning was his realization that any given motor ability is a distinct factor which may only relate to the performance of a specific part of the total activity performance. He argued the probable existence of many such factors and hypothesized that success in a sport or a particular activity within a sport relies on a combination of several such factors rather than any single factor of ability.

The growth of knowledge pertaining to the fundamental characteristics of motor learning was accompanied by an ever-increasing realization of the highly specific nature of motor skills. Fairclough (1952), in a study dealing with transfer in motor learning, wrote that motor skills are highly specific in their nature and that there are no general coordinations which transfer from task to task. Henry and Nelson (1956) also observed the high specificity characteristic of motor skills, for intercorrelations between these tasks occur only when there are obvious common elements. The authors conclude that one cannot measure motor ability through scores derived from performance on particular motor tasks since such measures fail to provide a valid estimate of learning aptitude. Ammons (1958) noted that the common elements which underlie the bilateral transfer of skill are largely confined to such nonspecific factors as prior experience, motivation, attention, and cogitive problem-solving abilities, rather than to any specific task-related factors.

Bachman (1961) observed an absence of correlation between individual differences in performance and learning abilities for two gross motor tasks which purportedly involved similar ability factors: the free-standing ladder climb and the stabilimeter balance. He argues that, since the high degree of specificity associated with the acquisition of motor skills virtually precludes the existence of a general factor of motor ability, the relationship observed between motor-ability test batteries and the acquisition of specific motor skills is due to motivational factors or biomechanical factors resulting from differences in body type rather than to differences in innate ability.

Fleishman (1964) employed factor analytic techniques to identify two broad domains of motor ability: the psychomotor, comprised of eleven discrete subabilities; and the gross motor, comprised of nine such abilities. The psychomotor abilities relate to proficiency in activities involving extrinsically-paced, highly speeded movements of the wrist, hand, and fingers; the gross motor abilities are central to skills involving intrinsically-paced movements of the trunk and limbs. Fleishman (1967) clearly differentiated the respective roles of abilities and skills in the learning process. He argued that abilities are more or less permanent behavioral traits which develop as a result of environmental and biological factors. Skills involve the application of one or more abilities in the performance of a particular task. Although Fleishman (1966) acknowledged that the initial learning of a motor task may involve factors different from those governing advanced levels of proficiency, and that motor skills are highly specific entities in and of themselves, he firmly stated that a subject's pretest abilities can interact significantly with the processes of motor learning.

Jones (1966) argued that the number of motor abilities may well be an infinite value since these factors are functions of the learner rather than the requirements of the task. Jones contended that ability factors are organized along physiological and behavioral lines and, therefore, cannot be measured adequately through testing. He argued that, given the high degree of specificity associated with motor skills, performance upon any given task reflects the organization of the task rather than that of the individual.

## Superdiagonal Form

Jones substantiated his position on the specificity of motor skills by citing the phenomenon of superdiagonal form observed in correlation matrices for motor performance measures. Since there is a diminishing ordinal relationship between increasingly distant sets of trials upon the same task, he contends that there is an ever-increasing level of specificity associated with acquisition of motor skill as learning proceeds from initial to advanced levels. Jones (1980) provides a practical example of the superdiagonal phenomenon in a study dealing with the acquisition of swimming skills. He makes three fundamental observations:

1. As students progressed to higher skill levels, their number diminished.
2. Students who attained the highest skill level (swimmer) required less time to complete each of the prerequisite courses (beginner, advanced-beginner, and intermediate) than those who failed to complete the swimmer requirement. Jones refers to this saving trend as sequential precession.
3. As the skill level increases, the degree of savings or sequential precession decreases. Although swimmers acquired the beginner skills in the least time, this saving progressively decreased for the advanced-beginner and intermediate skills. The farther the same students advanced in skill level, the smaller the advantage they enjoyed over students at the same level. He refers to this decrease in savings with increase in skill as diminishing returns.

Jones contends that while sequential precession and diminishing returns are independent factors, they can both be explained by the common phenomenon of increasing task specificity. In essence, the more advanced the level of skill, the more select it becomes in relation to the underlying abilities.

A further substantiation of the specificity of motor learning is provided by Welch and Henry (1971), who observe that the correlations between individual scores on adjacent trials were substantially uninfluenced by practice, but the interpolation of successively increasing numbers of trials between any pair of trials caused a progressive drop in the observed correlation between that pair of trials. It was also observed, however, that the interpolation of rest periods between the trials in which no practice was permitted also contributed to this effect of remoteness.

This latter observation casts some doubt upon the hypothesis that the decreasing correlation between increasingly separated trials is solely the result of a changing task-factor structure. The fact that the mere temporal separation of trials alone can result in a decreasing pattern of correlation between adjacent trials may well indicate that the super-diagonal form of a correlation matrix reflects the effects of practice distribution as well as changes in factor structure.

Thomas and Halliwell (1976) found that there generally tends to be a decreasing relationship between initial ability measures and criterion performance. This is particularly true when performance is extended over a long period of time and is characterized by a series of interpolated practice intervals, each separated by periods of rest. They observed such low correlations between initial trials and final trials for three different motor skills that the initial phases of motor learning must be essentially dependent upon factors basically unrelated to final performance. In fact, the prediction of final achievement from partial achievement was valid only after 95 percent of the task had been acquired. Predicated upon these findings, the authors conclude that in acquisition of motor skill the prediction of final achievement from initial performance constitutes an entirely unsatisfactory procedure.

A number of theorectical arguments have been advanced to explain this lack of relationship between inital and final performance. Kientzle (1949) theorizes that the superdiagonal phenomenon is attributable to the fact that practice changes the underlying abilities entering a task and that the relative contribution of any of these abilities to the variance of the task at any point in the learning process is dependent upon the number of trials rather than the amount of interpolated rest between trials.

This contention was at least partially substantiated by Fleishman and Rich (1963), who observed that the initial learning of a motor skill relied heavily upon the capacity to process visual information. Kinesthetic ability was critical in later learning. The attainment of advanced levels of proficiency was dependent upon the subject's ability to make the transition from visual to kinesthetic cues.

Ferguson (1956) hypothesized that the changing factor structure associated with increasing proficiency in motor learning resulted from the interaction between organizational and integrative reference variables with the fundamental motor ability factors. Although such reference variables have yet to be identified experimentally, Ferguson contends that it is their presence which accounts for the individual's capacity to meet the increasingly selective demands imposed during the course of learning.

Bilodeau and Bilodeau (1961) held that the phenomenon of superdiagonal form may be due to the accumulation of reactive inhibition during the course of practice. The progressively decreasing correlations between the first trial and successive trials are attributed to the growth of $I_R$ and its consequent proportionally increasing contribution to the variance of the task. It is argued that the growth of the $I_R$ increases stability and consequently decreases the communality between early and late performance upon the criterion task. The fact that the phenomenon of superdiagonal form persists even when trials are separated only by time casts considerable doubt upon the Bilodeau hypothesis since reactive inhibition is believed to dissipate over time.

Ammons (1952) theorized that practice distribution results in a pattern of increasing dissimilarity between succeedingly distant pairs of trials due to response generalization. In the case of skill acquisition, however, the converse of this position may well apply. The diminution in the communality of the variances of highly spaced trials is more likely to be due to increased specificity than to response generalization.

Buss (1973) wrote that abilities may actually be dynamic factors which are continually modified through interactions with the learning process, rather than comparatively stable behavioral traits. If this were true, any abilities which could be identified within the learner prior to acquisition would be radically altered following the acquisition of the criterion task. This would account for the decreasing correlation between performance upon the initial trial and upon succeedingly distant ones.

Although a variety of theoretical arguments have been advanced to explain the decreasing pattern of correlations between an initial measure and succeedingly distant measures of performance upon the same task, none has proven entirely satisfactory. The explanation of the phenomenon of superdiagonal form may well lie within the province of information theory—the increasing task specificity accompanying the growth of proficiency in motor performance could conceivably result from decreasing the uncertainty associated with the initial phase of acquisition. In other words, the apparent changes in the factor structure which distinguish later learning from early learning could be the result of an increasing degree of relative redundancy during the later phases of skill acquisition. This argument concerning the role of uncertainty in the initial phases of motor learning is in part substantiated by the findings of Bilodeau (1957), who observed far greater variability in the performance of the novice than in that of the highly skilled subject. Eckert (1974) also observed that variability of response is greatest during the early stages of learning and during periods of increasing complexity.

### Limitations of Testing Procedures

The problem of identifying and measuring pretask abilities presents one of the most difficult obstacles in understanding the place of individual differences in motor learning. Although tests which accurately measure factors of motor ability have yet to be developed, Guilford (1965) cautioned that no one test can ever be a wholly unadulterated measure of a basic ability or behavioral trait. No test can be completely confined to the measurement of a single factor. In addition, no test is perfectly reliable; there will always be some variability in its internal consistency. Kleinman (1976), for example, found the reliability of the

Metheny-Johnson Test to be .63 (n=369), and each of its four subtests, .70 to .25.

The problem of validity is another major factor in clarifying the role of basic abilities in the acquisition of motor skill. Since the concept of predictive validity rests upon the correlation between the predictive index and the criterion measure, the high degree of task-specific variance associated with motor skills greatly reduces the amount of common variance which could be shared with any predictive measure. Although this high specificity places severe constraints upon the accuracy of any predictive index, it is a generally accepted principle that a baseline measure with low predictive validity is more desirable than a situation in which no predictive indices exist. What is the minimum acceptable value for a validity coefficient? Since validity is a relative rather than an absolute concept, the best value is often simply the highest correlation attainable under a given set of circumstances. Frequently, the only constraint placed upon the magnitude of a validity coefficient is that it must be statistically significant.

*Task Taxonomy*

Yet another factor limiting the precise prediction of attainable motor learning level from pretask abilities pertains to the broader issue of task taxonomy. Fitts (1964) writes that motor tasks may be classified according to properties of complexity, coherence, continuity, and pacing. Complex tasks involve not only a greater number of abilities than simple tasks, but they also provide for a correspondingly greater number of possible permutations and interactions between these abilities and other task-related factors. Just as the outcome of a recipe for some culinary delight cannot be adequately described in terms of the properties of each individual ingredient, so performance upon a complex motor task could not be predicted in total, even if it were theoretically possible to identify all of its constituent elements prior to acquisition.

The coherence of a task relates to its internal consistency or relative redundancy. The more coherent a task, the greater the similarity between its initial phases and its final phases. Performance on highly redundant tasks such as pursuit-rotor tracking, for example, should be more readily predictable from a prior knowledge of pretask abilities than performance upon tasks which are low in redundancy. Performance upon tasks which reflect marked discontinuities or periodicities in their nature is more difficult to predict than performance upon continuous tasks. Even though the constituent ability constructs of a task may be identified prior to learning, marked fluctuations in its temporal and spatial patterning greatly complicate the problem of prediction. The sequence in which the abilities are applied, as well as variations in their respective requisite amplitudes, are vital elements in the motor learning process. Thus, the degree of accuracy with which one can predict the final outcome of a situation, based upon some prior knowledge of the constituent elements of that situation, is contingent upon the degree of consistency governing the relationship between those elements.

Lastly, the pacing of a task is a factor limiting the accuracy of prediction. Extrinsically-paced tasks are dependent upon different ability factors than tasks which are intrinsically-paced. If one were concerned, for example, with predicting success in learning the forehand stroke in tennis, the performance of the skill by volleying against a wall (intrinsic pacing) would be a less valid predictor of criterion achievement than performance of the skill by returning balls delivered by an automatic serving machine (extrinsic pacing). If a predictive index is to be valid, its temporal pacing must closely approximate that of the criterion measure.

Billing (1980) writes that the complexity of the information processed in the learning and performance of a motor skill is a critical parameter of task taxonomy. Such complexity is a function of the number of responses required in the execution of a given skill and the speed and accuracy with which they must be elicited. The author contends that a taxonomy of motor tasks should account for such perceptual factors as the intensity, duration, and number of stimuli; the nature of the information feedback (terminal or concurrent); and the speed and precision of the decision-making processes required in the execution of the skill.

### Human Factor

A final factor limiting the predictive accuracy of motor performance from pretask abilities pertains to the nature of motor learning itself. Fitts (1962) proposed three stages in the acquisition of complex motor skills: cognition, fixation, and automation. The initial stage, cognition, involves direct cortical mediation and is dependent upon the presence of perceptual, verbal, and visual abilities. (Demonstration and explanation are critical at this level.) The second phase, fixation, is characterized by the gradual diminution of active cortical mediation and the consequent shift in dependence from extrinsic to intrinsic cues. During the fixation phase, the regulation and mediation of the activity are progressively relegated to the lower centers of the brain where movements are effected in response to perceived changes in pressure and direction. In the final phase of skill acquisition, the stage of automation, information generated by the proprioceptive feedback from the muscles, joints, and tendons is processed by lower centers in the nervous system concerned with the servoregulatory control of stereotyped patterns of movement.

Fitts' three-stage model may well be a valid theoretical explanation of the changing factor structure associated with the growth of proficiency in motor learning and the resultant phenomenon of superdiagonal correlation. Current research findings concerning the structure and function of the motor system (Eccles, 1969, 1973; Gawronski, 1971, Granit, 1970; Kornhuber, 1974) mostly substantiate Fitts' statements about the respective roles of the various nervous system segments during the different stages of motor learning. (For an in-depth discussion, see Chapter 6.)

It is possible to identify behavioral traits which are in varying degree common to a number of motor skills. Although the correlation between performance on a particular task and a given ability factor may be low, such relationships do in fact exist. The major problems confronting researchers studying the role of individual differences in motor learning pertain to the identification and objective measurement of these factors of motor ability and to their respective interactions with such conditions of motor learning as distribution of practice, task taxonomy, and level of learning.

### Applications to Teaching

Of all the research on the role of ability factors, it is the work of Fleishman which most readily lends itself to practical application in the teaching of motor skills. Through his discovery of two distinct domains of motor abilities, the gross motor and the psychomotor, Fleishman (1966, 1967) provided insight into the factors which underlie proficiency in the acquisition and performance of different types of motor tasks.

The gross motor domain is comprised of nine independent abilities, four of which involve the factor of strength.

1. "Explosive strength" is central to the performance of skills involving sudden rapid bursts of muscular energy against forces which offer less than maximal resistance. Kicking, throwing, jumping, and all forms of striking activities (tennis, baseball, badminton, squash) are all dependent upon the factor of explosive strength. Other examples of the function of this ability factor are the start of a race or the charge of football linemen forward from the line of scrimmage when the ball is passed from center.

2. "Dynamic strength" (known also as "muscular endurance") is vital to activities which involve sustained or repeated muscular contractions. As in the case of explosive strength, dynamic strength is called for in situations which require less than maximal effort. The most

common activities requiring dynamic strength are calisthenic-type exercises (push-ups, pull-ups, dips on the parallel bars, chins). Dynamic strength is also critical in many gymnastic movements, particularly those involving "held" positions.

3. "Static strength" is defined as the capacity to exert an all-out muscular contraction against maximal resistance. The muscular force exerted is of such magnitude that it can be neither sustained nor repeated. Probably the best example of static strength in motor performance is competitive weight lifting: the performer attempts to lift the greatest amount of weight for a brief period of time.

4. "Abdominal strength" is a form of dynamic strength confined to the abdominal area and is central to such activities as sit-ups and leg raises. (In the latter case, the abdominal muscles serve primarily as stabilizers.)

In addition to the four strength factors, Fleishman identified two factors related to flexibility.

5. "Extent flexibility" is measured in terms of the range of motion at the hip joint. The subject is required to move the trunk from the deepest forward bend to the deepest back bend (extreme flexion to extreme extension). The greater the total range of motion, the higher the subject's rating. Extent flexibility is an important requisite in such activities as gymnastics, diving, and dance.

6. "Dynamic flexibility" pertains to the resiliency of the muscles in relation to their ability to recover rapidly from stretch. It is measured in terms of the subject's capacity to make a series of rapidly repeated, bobbing motions, going from full flexion to full extension of the trunk. Physiologically, there is danger of muscular injury through the intervention of the myotatic stretch reflex (the rapid stretching of the muscle reflexively causes that same muscle to contract). Because of this danger and the limited applicability of dynamic flexibility, it is suggested that this particular factor can be eliminated from an ability-testing program.

It may be said that these six factors are central to such intrinsically-paced activities as gymnastics, diving, and weight lifting.

The three remaining gross motor ability constructs are applicable to a broader range of activities.

7. "Gross body coordination" is a broad ability construct which entails an individual's capacity to make coordinated movements of the arms and legs while the body is in motion. This ability construct is central to such diverse skills as throwing a running pass in football, dribbling in basketball, and executing a forehand stroke in tennis.

8. "Gross body equilibrium" is defined as the capacity to resist forces

which throw the body off balance. It is critical to the successful execution of skills involving rapid changes in the direction of bodily movements, such as a runningback in a football game employing evasive movements in broken field running. This ability is also important in the execution of many gymnastic movements, particularly those required in free exercise and balance beam routines.

9. "Stamina" is most commonly referred to as cardiorespiratory endurance and is essential in all activities involving sustained levels of cardiovascular stress (e.g., distance running). Current research evidence indicates that this ability can be developed through appropriate conditioning programs, even during later life.

In addition to the nine gross motor ability factors, Fleishman identified eleven psychomotor abilities. The major difference between these two domains is in the nature of the abilities' temporal regulation within each. Gross motor abilities are usually central to activities which are intrinsically-paced; the timing of the response is solely at the discretion of the learner. The execution of a gymnastic routine, weight lifting, and diving are all examples of activities dependent upon gross motor abilities. Responses which are dependent upon psychomotor abilities, in contrast, are largely under the control of extrinsic temporal factors. Since most of the psychomotor abilities tend to underlie behavioral responses which must be rapidly executed in answer to extrinsic cues, they are particularly important in the performance of team sport activities where the pace of the game is frequently determined by the strategies and tactics of the opposition.

1. "Control precision" is defined by Fleishman as the capacity to make controlled, but not overcontrolled movements of large muscle groups, particularly under speeded conditions. This ability is central to all movements involving follow-through. Throwing, kicking, and striking (as in tennis, baseball, and golf) are all dependent upon this factor. Subjects who are deficient in this ability tend to manifest overcontrolled, choppy movement patterns.

2. "Multi-limb coordination" (which has little application to the teaching of sport skills) concerns the capacity to make coordinated movements of the arms and legs while in a stationary position. Playing a grand organ or driving a motor vehicle with a standard transmission are good examples of activities dependent upon multi-limb coordination.

3. "Response orientation" is an extremely broad factor which is critical to success in many of the team sports. It involves the capacity to select the appropriate movement in response to the correct stimulus under highly speeded conditions, i.e., the capacity

to make the right move at the right time quickly. Just as the mastery of the basic skills is essential to developing proficiency in any sports activity, the learner's capacity for response orientation can distinguish a mediocre performer from one who excels.

4. "Reaction time" (of limited value in the acquisition of skill) merely represents the speed with which an individual can respond to a stimulus. The course of action is predetermined and there is no decision-making involved. This factor comes into play during the start of a race. The contestant elicits a predetermined response (leaving the starting block) to a particular stimulus (the sound of the gun).

5. "Rate control" is one of the broadest psychomotor abilities and involves the capacity to track an object whose speed and direction are continually changing. This ability is particularly important in a defensive player. (His capacity to "stick like a shadow" to his man is a function of this factor.) Rate control is important in any defensive game situation, such as preparing to return a serve in tennis or badminton, or tracking a fly in baseball.

6. "Speed of arm movement" involves the capacity to make a discrete rapid movement of the arms. Accuracy is not an important aspect in this ability, which underlies such movements as a defensive player's raising arms to block a shot by the offense in a basketball game or a boxer's raising arms in a defensive stance.

7. "Manual dexterity" is critical to success in the ball sports. The ability is defined as the capacity to manipulate large objects with the hands under speeded conditions. It is used in all activities involving catching, throwing, and the use of striking implements, such as bats and rackets.

8. "Finger dexterity" has little relevance to the acquisition of sport skills and is primarily confined to the manipulation of small objects, such as the tools used in watch repair.

9. "Arm-hand steadiness" is that which enables an individual to make precise positioning movements of the arm and hand under conditions where speed is not a critical factor. This ability is important in such activities as archery, dance, and free exercise routines in gymnastics.

10. "Wrist-finger speed," also known as "tapping ability," is of limited value in the acquisiton of motor skills.

11. "Aiming," or eye-hand coordination, is central to all skills which involve throwing or projecting an object toward a target (the jump shot in basketball or the serve in tennis).

Although Fleishman's work encompasses the psychomotor and gross motor domains, it is by no means an exhaustive taxonomy of human motor ability. It does, however, provide a framework within which the teacher of motor skills can operate more effectively. These ability factors provide a basis for assessing individual differences in capacity for learning different types of motor skills prior to their actual acquisition. With this knowledge, the physical educator can plan programs of instruction as well as remediation.

Individual differences in ability are important aspects in planning such programs, but the nature of the learning tasks employed is often overlooked. Billing (1975) provides a system for classifying complex motor skills based upon broad theoretical guidelines.

1.  The nature of the physical act itself. Motor skills are divided into four subgroups: manipulative, ballistic, body oriented, and object oriented. Manipulative skills stress form and accuracy; ballistic skills emphasize speed and power. Body-oriented skills focus on the precise control of bodily movements (e.g., dance, gymnastics, diving); object-oriented skills focus on the tracking of an object whose speed and trajectory are dependent upon extrinsic forces (e.g. hockey, tennis, baseball).

2.  The nature of the opponent interaction. This category is divided into two subgroups: autonomous skills and reactive skills. In the former, the participant is free to set his or her own pace and direction of performance (e.g., bowling, golf). In the latter, the responses of the performer are directly affected by those of the opponent (e.g., basketball, soccer).

3.  The units of competition—do they entail individual or team participation? Individual sports are defined as activities in which the performer receives no assistance or cooperation from another participant during the entire course of the activity. (This classification is valid even though individual scores may be summed to determine team standing.) In team sports, at least two performers must engage in the activity as a cooperative unit (e.g., tennis doubles).

4.  The continuousness or intermittence of the time component. In continuous activities, play proceeds for an uninterrupted interval until points are scored, an object or player transcends the boundaries of the playing area, or some form of foul is committed (e.g., hockey, basketball, soccer). An intermittent activity is characterized by a series of attempts, separated by time or rest intervals (e.g., shot put, high jump).

5.  The nature of the learning environment—constant or varied. A constant environment is characterized by exact markings or definitions of play area or surfaces (e.g., a baseball diamond, a football

field, or a basketball court). A varied environment often entails natural terrain and will change from place to place (e.g., cross-country skiing, running a marathon).

Subject ability and the interaction between the factors of task taxonomy are critical considerations in the planning of an instructional program. In order to facilitate the acquisition of a motor skill and ensure that a reasonable level of proficiency is attained, it is essential that the learner possess sufficient levels of the abilities requisite to the execution of a given criterion task. This end can be accomplished through a knowledge of the nature of the learning task and the abilities and interests of the learner.

The use of pretask ability factors can augment the instructional program, but caution must be employed when utilizing ability grouping. Frequently, subjects of low ability are stigmatized and a negative effect on the student's self-concept results. When students are grouped according to ability, the composition of each group should change with each activity under study. Ability level should be regarded as a factor which is relative to the taxonomical characteristics of a given criterion task rather than as an absolute entity. No group should be viewed as being either "good" or "bad." Although the instructor should make every attempt to correct the students' weaknesses, he must also strive to maximize their particular strengths and to build their confidence.

Whether the performance of individuals whose initial ability levels differ will become more or less alike after equal amounts of practice is another issue. This problem is compounded by motivational factors because subjects of lower ability are most likely to encounter high levels of frustration during the acquisition of a given task. Although there is little a teacher can do to influence directly a learner's ability level prior to the acquisition of the criterion task, there are many motivational techniques which can be employed to compensate for such differences. Whenever possible, students should be allowed to learn at their own pace and their progress should be assessed in terms of their individual capacities rather than in comparison to the other members of the class. It may often be necessary for the teacher to structure the learning environment so that each student may proceed in an incremental fashion, i.e., each unit in the instruction process is tailored to the capacity of the learner. Such an approach would allow the more skilled individuals to proceed in larger increments and at the same time provide individuals of lower ability with a structured framework in which small but significant advances can be achieved.

Although controversy over the fundamental nature of human abilities continues (are they acquired or innate), there is general consensus that individual differences in ability levels prior to the acquisition of the criterion task limit the learning process. Perhaps one of the most significant functions of ability factors in motor learning is their facilitating role in processing various types of sensory input. Since an ability may be viewed as a capacity for processing a specific type of information (verbal, visual, kinesthetic), individual differences in the levels of these abilities can exert a profound effect upon the subjects' response to specific methods of instruction in the acquisition of a given criterion task.

Among individuals with a facility for processing verbal information, there are those who will respond well to written instruction and others who will profit more from the spoken word. A learner with a facility for processing visual input will profit most from instructional techniques which emphasize illustration and demonstration; those with a facility for processing verbal information will profit most from spoken or written instructions. In order to attain optimal learning, the method of instruction employed should be geared to the most pronounced sensory capacities of the subject.

*References*

Ammons, R.B. "Relationship of Motivation and Method of Testing to Distribution of Practice Phenomena in Rotary Pursuit." *Quarterly Journal of Experimental Psychology, 4* (1952), 155–164.

––––––. "Le Mouvement." *In* G.S. and J.P. Seward (eds.), *Current Psychological Issues.* New York: Holt, 1958.

Bachman, J. "Specificity versus Generality in Learning and Performing Two Large Muscle Motor Tasks." *Research Quarterly, 32* (1961), 3–11.

Bechtoldt, H.P. "Motor Abilities in Studies of Motor Learning." *In* L.E. Smith (ed.), *Psychology of Motor Learning.* Chicago: The Athletic Institute, 1970.

Billing, J. "A Taxonomy of Sport Forms." *Annual Proceedings of the National College Physical Education Association, 78* (1975), 34–39.

––––––. "An Overview of Task Complexity." *Motor Skills: Theory Into Practice, 4* (1980), 18–23.

Bilodeau, E. "The Relationship Between a Relatively Complex Motor Skill and Its Components." *American Journal of Psychology, 70* (1957), 49–55.

–––––– and I.M. "Motor Skills Learning." *Annual Review of Psychology, 12* (1961), 243–280.

Brace, D.K. *Measuring Motor Ability* . New York: Barnes, 1926.

———. "Studies in Motor Learning of Gross Bodily Motor Skills." *Research Quarterly, 17* (1946), 242–253.

Buss, A.R. "Learning Transfer and Ability Factors: A Multivariate Model." *Psychological Bulletin, 80* (1973), 106–112.

Eccles, J.C. "The Dynamic Loop Hypothesis of Movement Control." *In* K.N. Leibovic (ed.), *Information Processing in the Nervous System.* New York: Springer-Verlag, 1969.

———. *The Understanding of the Brain.* New York: McGraw-Hill, 1973.

Eckert, H.M. "Variability in Skill Acquisition." *Child Development, 45* (1974), 487–489.

Fairclough, R.N. "Transfer of Motivated Improvements in Speed of Reaction and Movements." *Research Quarterly, 23* (1952), 20–28.

Ferguson, G.A. "On Transfer and the Abilities of Man." *Canadian Journal of Psychology, 10* (1956), 121–131.

Fitts, P.M. "Factors in Complex Skill Training." *In* R. Glaser (ed.), *Training Research and Education.* Pittsburgh: Pittsburgh University Press, 1962.

———. "Perceptual-Motor Skill Learning." *In* A. Melton (ed.), *Categories of Human Learning.* New York: Academic Press, 1964.

Fleishman, E.A. *The Structure and Measurement of Physical Fitness.* Englewood Cliffs, NJ: Prentice-Hall, 1964.

———. "Human Abilities and the Acquisition of Skill." *In* E.A. Bilodeau (ed.), *Acquisition of Skill.* New York: Academic Press, 1966.

———. "Individual Differences and Motor Learning." *In* R. Gagné (ed.), *Learning and Individual Differences.* Columbus, Ohio: Merrill, 1967.

——— and S. Rich. "The Role of Kinesthetic and Spatial-Visual Ability in Perceptual-Motor Learning." *Journal of Experimental Psychology, 56* (1963), 6–11.

Gawronski, R. *Bionics.* New York and Amsterdam: Elsevier, 1971.

Gire, E. and A. Espenschade. "The Relationship Between Measures of Motor Educability and the Learning of Specific Motor Skills." *Research Quarterly, 13* (1942), 43–56.

Granit, R. *The Basis of Motor Control.* New York: Academic Press, 1970.

Guilford, J. P. *Fundamental Statistics in Psychology and Education.* 4th ed. New York: McGraw-Hill, 1965.

Henry, F.M. and G.A. Nelson. "Age Differences and Inter-Relationships Between Skill Learning in Gross Motor Performance of Ten and Fifteen Year Old Boys." *Research Quarterly, 27* (1956), 162–175.

Johnson, G.B. "Physical Skill Tests for Sectioning Classes Into Homogeneous Units." *Research Quarterly, 3* (1932), 128–134.

Jones, M.B. "Individual Differences." *In* E.A. Bilodeau (ed.), *Acquisition of Skill.* New York: Academic Press, 1966.

————. "Sequential Precession and Diminishing Returns in the Acquisition of a Motor Skill." *Journal of Motor Behavior, 12* (1980), 69–73.

Kientzle, N.J. "Ability Patterns Under Distributed Practice." *Journal of Experimental Psychology, 39* (1949), 532– 537.

Kleinman, M. "The Predictive Validity of the Metheny-Johnson Test." Paper presented at the meeting of the Eastern District Association of the American Association for Health, Physical Education and Recreation, Mount Pocono, Pa., March 1976.

Kornhuber, H.H. "Cerebral Cortex, Cerebellum and Basal Ganglia: An Introduction to Their Motor Functions." *In* F. Schmitt and F.G. Worden (eds.), *The Neurosciences.* Cambridge, Mass.: MIT Press, 1974.

McCauley, M., R. Kennedy, and A. Bittner. "Development of Performance Evaluation Tests for Environmental Research (PETER): Time Estimation." *Perceptual and Motor Skills, 51* (1980), 655–665.

McCloy, C.H. "The Measurement of General Motor Capacity and General Motor Ability." *Research Quarterly Supplement, 5* (1934), 46–61.

————. "An Analytical Study of the Stunt Type Test As a Measure of Motor Educability." *Research Quarterly, 7* (1937), 46–55.

McCraw, L.W. "A Factor Analysis of Motor Learning." *Research Quarterly, 20* (1949), 162–175.

Metheny, E. "Studies of the Johnson Test As a Test of Motor Educability." *Research Quarterly, 9* (1938), 105–114.

Noble, C.E. "Age, Race, and Sex in the Learning and Performance of Psychomotor Skills." *In* R.T. Osborne, C.E. Noble, and N. Weyl (eds.), *Human Variation: The Biopsychology of Age, Race, and Sex.* New York: Academic Press, 1978.

Thomas, J.R. and W. Halliwell. "Individual Differences in Motor Skill Acquisition." *Journal of Motor Behavior, 8* (1976), 89–99.

Welch, M. and F.M. Henry. "Individual Differences in Various Parameters of Motor Learning." *Journal of Motor Behavior, 3* (1971), 78–96.

# CHAPTER 8

# Information Theory and Knowledge of Results

DURING THE FIRST HALF of this century, the scientific study of human learning was dominated by two opposing theoretical positions, respondent and operant conditioning. (See Chapter 2) The older of these two schools, respondent or Type I, is rooted in the theoretical traditions of Pavlov's classical conditioning. Its advocates argue that all learning is the result of the paired association between a stimulus and a response in close temporal contiguity. Unfortunately, these respondent theorists have shown little interest in the intrinsic mechanisms which could account for the factors underlying an individual's capacity to associate two events contiguously. They have never concerned themselves with such fundamental questions as how these associative processes function and why certain responses, for example reflexes, are better conditioned through contiguous association than are more complex forms of behavior.

Although theories favoring contiguous stimulus-response association as the central element in learning were the first to evolve, operant or Type II conditioning theory has come to predominate much of contemporary learning research. Operant theorists contend that the critical element in learning is the consequences of the response itself (the reinforcement) rather than the bond between a stimulus and a response. Although operant principles currently enjoy successful application in such diverse areas as education, behavior therapy, and animal training, proponents of this school do not concern themselves with such fundamental theoretical issues as how and why reinforcement exerts its effects.

### Control System Models

It is this apparent lack of theoretical sophistication in Type I and Type II conditioning principles that has resulted in the development of alternative views of the factors underlying learning. Opponents of respondent and operant conditioning principles argue that behavior and learning are the consequences of the direct dynamic sensory effects of the response itself (feedback) rather than the consequences of the aftereffects of the response (reinforcement). Smith (1970) regards behavior as a self-governed series of motor-sensory processes which rely upon information feedback concerning the reciprocal interactions between motor functions and sensory input. Each response alters the stimulus input, resulting in a modification of the following response. A student in a physical education class learning to perform a headstand kicks off the ground too forcefully during the first attempt and, as a result, overbalances and lands flat on his back. Based upon the sensory input obtained from this attempt, the student applies less force on the next trial and underbalances, landing on his toes. Eventually, based upon the information feedback obtained from preceding trials, the student will modulate his response through neural processes and acquire the task.

Smith contends that all coordinated motor activity is a function of closed-loop processes involving the temporal combination and coordination of postural, transport, and manipulative movement components which are integrated by the inflow of response-produced feedback. Such feedback may be exteroceptive, static, or dynamic. Exteroceptive feedback consists of visual and auditory information and is most important during the initial phases of skill acquisition. As proficiency develops, however, there is an increasing dependence upon proprioceptive feedback in the regulation and control of coordinated patterns of complex movements. Dynamic feedback represents the continuous flow of exteroceptive and proprioceptive information generated as a consequence of the temporal and spatial changes occurring during the course of the actual execution of a movement. Static feedback represents the aftereffects of a response on the environment (the knowledge of results).

In an activity such as bowling, for example, the dynamic feedback arises from the actions associated with the approach and delivery of the ball; the static feedback arises from the environmental consequences of the movement (e.g., the number of pins knocked down). Dynamic feedback integrates factors of space, time, and force, and is therefore more essential in the control of movement than static feedback, which is primarily confined to the guidance of a movement. The temporal patterning of dynamic feedback information is so precise and highly specific, however, that even minor alterations or delays in its processing can result in severe disruption of performance.

Feedback is also essential in motor memory since the degree to which a given movement is retained is dependent upon its direct sensory effects. Although the interval between a movement and its sensory feedback will vary from skill to skill, the precise duration of this interval will be constant for a particular movement. It is these specific temporal characteristics of a skill, along with other spatial and force-related feedback information, which are retained and enable the learner to program a motor memory store which can ultimately serve as a predictive feedforward control process for the anticipation of future movements.

According to the closed-loop theory of motor control, the greater the degree of self-regulated control over sensory feedback, the greater the potential scope of learning and the greater the speed of acquisition. Conversely, the greater the learner's dependence upon such external environmental factors as reinforcement and stimulus-response contiguity, the slower and narrower the scope of learning and the more unstable and inconsistent the learned response. The smooth coordination of the diverse bodily activities required in the learning and performance of complex motor skills is possible only through the integrative effects of feedback upon the motor regulatory process.

Smith's views are rooted in information theory or cybernetics, which is concerned with the field of control and communication in machines and in living organisms. Information feedback plays a central role in cybernetics and is defined by Wiener (1948) as the information resulting from the difference between the pattern of action desired and the pattern actually obtained. The information concerning the magnitude of this difference serves as an additional stimulus input to the regulatory mechanism (the nervous system in the case of learning and behavior) which effects dynamic adjustments, resulting in a diminution of the discrepancy between the ongoing pattern of activity and the pattern desired. Through practice and continual response modification based upon information feedback, the criterion task is ultimately attained. Since feedback is critical in the execution of any activity which requires continual regulation and adjustment, fluctuations in either its amount or its temporal patterning can result in severe disruption of the ongoing activity.

An insufficient amount of feedback will severely hamper the execution of an activity, as in the attempt to acquire a complex task by trial and error. Assume that an individual with no knowledge of music is seated at a piano and told to perform a classical sonata perfectly and from memory, or that someone with no skill in gymnastics is led to a set of parallel bars and told to improvise a competitive gymnastic routine. The prospects for success in either case are exceedingly dim. Since the response-produced feedback fails to provide the learner with sufficient information concerning the correctness of his response, the same errors are continually repeated.

An excess amount of feedback, particularly when temporally delayed, can prove equally harmful to the regulation of the activity. A prime mechanical example of the counterproductive effects of excessive amounts of temporally delayed feedback is the unfortunate individual riding in a railroad car with a malfunctioning thermostat. Since the action of the thermostat lags considerably behind the conditions prevailing in the car, the temperature is allowed to rise to excessively uncomfortable levels before the heating element is turned off. Since the thermostat continues to lag well behind the true conditions in the car, the temperature will fall to excessively low levels before the heating element is turned back on. If this situation is allowed to continue, the swings in temperature will grow increasingly more extreme, vacillating radically between high and low.

Excessive bursts of feedback set the system off-balance and, in turn, effect an overcompensation in the opposite direction, setting the system into oscillation. A physiological example of the deleterious effects of excessive bursts of feedback can be found in cerebellar or purpose tremor. The individual afflicted with this condition is unable to control reaching or manipulative movements to such an extent that any attempt to perform a controlled act results in a series of extreme oscillations about the desired goal. He cannot drink a glass of water without spilling its contents, for he will continually overshoot and undershoot the area of the mouth when attempting to bring the glass to the lips. The greatest danger inherent in excessive amounts of feedback lies in the possibility of sending the system into violent oscillation while attempting to hunt for the appropriate response. The consequences of such extreme swings are invariably destructive to the system.

### Feedback and Knowledge of Results

Although controversy exists regarding the precise role of feedback in learning and performance, advances in neurophysiology and information theory provide abundant evidence of its critical function in the regulation and control of biological as well as mechanical systems. There are a number of factors which hinder the study of the functions of feedback in motor learning, but problems of definition, task taxonomy, and the learning-performance distinction are the primary sources of confusion. Bilodeau (1966) writes that the term "knowledge of results," or KR, often used synonymously with feedback, is particularly confusing since it only refers to the amount of extrinsic information a subject receives concerning the accuracy of his response. It does not consider any intrinsic processes which involve the perception and interpretation of such information.

Newell (1976) distinguishes between the two by defining knowledge of results as some type of information or score which is presented to the performer either verbally or mechanically during the course of acquisition and is the representation of the outcome of a movement. This score may entail a simple right or wrong or a statement reflecting the degree of error in the response. Feedback, in contrast, is defined as the sum of all the perceived aftereffects of the movement itself and involves visual, auditory, tactual, and kinesthetic sensory input. Since knowledge of results is confined primarily to verbal information, it is far better suited to experimental manipulation and control than the general phenomenon of information feedback. Unfortunately, despite attempts to clarify the respective roles of information feedback and knowledge of results in motor learning, these terms are still often used interchangeably. The problems encountered in the area of definition of terms are further compounded by the nature of the criterion task employed in any given study. Discrete tasks, such as lever positioning, are characterized by the presence of discernible intervals between each succeeding trial. Tasks such as tracking are continuous in nature with no perceptible intertrial interval. Since knowledge of results has been defined as information representing the outcome of a movement, it is far more applicable to the acquisition of discrete tasks (due to the presence of the intertrial interval within which such information can be provided) than it is to the acquisition of continuous tasks.

### Learning and Performance

A final issue which confounds the study of the role of feedback in motor learning pertains to the learning-performance distinction. Fleishman (1967) writes that although verbal and cognitive abilities appear to be important during the initial phases of motor learning, the importance diminishes as proficiency develops since there is an increasing dependence upon motor ability factors in the performance of the task following its acquisition. The early phases of motor learning are characterized by wide fluctuations in the precision of the desired response, and a great deal of adjustment and adaptation are required on behalf of the learner. Because verbal information is particularly valuable during this phase of acquisition, knowledge of results in the form of verbal feedback is most effective since the appropriate modifications in response require cognitive as well as motoric adaptations. The processing of this verbal information involves reasoning and decision-making. As proficiency is developed, however, the degree to which the desired response must be adjusted becomes considerably more refined and there is a marked shift toward increased dependence upon regulatory processess which require a steady flow of kinesthetic feedback and function in an automatic fashion without the need for conscious regulation. While the learning of a motor task depends upon verbal factors, its performance apparently does not.

Whenever an individual is lifting, throwing, or exerting any type of muscular force, there is a continual stream of feedback flowing in from the periphery, conveying information concerning the degree to which the task has been completed at any given point in time. The growth of proficiency in any skilled performance is attributed to the learner's capacity to process feedback information and thus systematically reduce the discrepancy between the movement outcome desired and the one ultimately attained. If the desired movement entails hitting a target with a thrown object, the feedback conveys information about the degree to which each throw is off its mark. Proficiency grows as this gap is narrowed. The old adage, "practice makes perfect," is in reality predicated upon the fact that learning is the result of practice which is accompanied by information feedback, which is itself initially reinforced by the presentation of knowledge of results.

### Feedback Variables

Feedback is a vital factor in the regulation and control of behavior, exerting its effects in a number of ways. It may be classified as positive or negative, continuous or intermittent, concurrent (dynamic) or terminal (static). Positive feedback results in the perpetuation of the prevailing conditions no matter if they are environmental, biological, or behavioral. Examples of positive feedback can be found in a nuclear chain reaction or in the more familiar situation of adding fuel to a fire. There are many pathological conditions in the physiological realm (e.g., hypertension and hypoglycemia), which result from a breakdown in homeostatic regulation, and, if left unchecked, tend to self-perpetuate with increasing severity, inevitably proving fatal to the organism.

An example of the deleterious effects of positive feedback in the behavioral realm is a verbal disagreement arising between a player and an official during the course of a game. The player, believing the official's decision to be incorrect, is angered and responds to the call in a flagrantly abusive manner. The player's actions, in turn, anger the official, who reacts in a hostile and belligerent way, further exciting the player. Clearly, if this situation is allowed to continue unabated, the level of hostility will escalate, possibly culminating in physical injury to the parties involved.

Negative feedback reverses the prevailing conditions in a given situation. One of the most common examples of a negative feedback device is in the room thermostat which raises the temperature when it falls below a certain point and shuts the heat off when it rises above a predetermined point. Negative feedback is critical in the maintenance and regulation of any mechanical, biological, or behavioral activity. The entire concept of homeostasis is dependent upon a series of negative feedback loops which keep biological processes within given limits.

Negative feedback is of particular consequence in motor learning since coordinated movement patterns are dependent upon the alternate contraction and relaxation of antagonistic muscle groups. Specialized nerve receptors are located in the muscles and tendons and mediate muscular activity through a network of feedback loops. A muscle spindle exerts negative feedback control over the muscle to which it is joined, at the same time exerting positive feedback control over its antagonistic muscle. If a muscle is suddenly stretched, tension on the muscle spindle is increased, causing the spindle to exert a negative feedback response which facilitates contraction of that muscle while simultaneously inhibiting contraction (positive feedback) in the antagonistic muscle. This reciprocal innervation effected by the muscle spindle is the physical basis of information feedback which governs the maintenance of posture below the level of consciousness.

In addition to its behavioral consequences, feedback can also be classified in terms of the temporal patterning with which it is received. Continuous feedback provides the learner with an unbroken stream of information through the entire duration of a particular activity. Intermittent feedback, in contrast, is provided only during discrete intervals. Continuous feedback is characteristic of the proprioceptive information generated during the course of the execution of a movement; knowledge of results is representative of intermittent feedback.

Robb (1972) redefined the concept of continuous and intermittent feedback by proposing the terms concurrent (dynamic) and terminal (static) feedback. According to Robb, concurrent feedback is central in complex behavior and is exemplified by the continuous stream of visual and proprioceptive information generated during the actual execution of the task. Terminal feedback, on the other hand, pertains to the knowledge of results obtained by the learner upon the completion of a task.

In performing the jump shot in basketball, for example, the proprioceptive, visual, and auditory stimuli which impinge upon the learner during the act of shooting constitute the concurrent feedback; the knowledge of the ultimate success or failure of the attempt, the terminal feedback. Concurrent feedback is critical in eliciting and regulating the appropriate subroutines which interact in the execution of a complex task. Terminal feedback functions much as does reinforcement. Reinforcement is typically associated with such simple discrete forms of behavior as a rat's pressing a bar or a pigeon's pecking a key for a pellet of food. Terminal feedback occurs, however, at the conclusion of any behavioral act, regardless of the complexity of its nature, and provides the learner with information concerning the degree of success or failure encountered in its performance. Terminal feedback is, in essence, a form of reinforcement which exerts its effects by providing the learner with information, as opposed to reducing some physiological drive.

### Open- and Closed-Loop Processes

Although cybernetic theories currently enjoy increasing application in the study of human learning and behavior, operant conditioning principles still retain a formidable position in learning research. In an attempt to clarify the theoretical controversy between these two opposing views, Adams (1971) hypothesized two types of behavior, open-loop and closed-loop, to demonstrate that information feedback plays a central role in all forms of learning.

Open-loop behavior is best characterized by motor responses which are elicited by the firing of a preprogramed pattern of neurons. The response is stereotyped in that, once initiated, it proceeds in a predetermined fashion despite variations in the prevailing environmental conditions (as a traffic light which alternates between red and green in a fixed pattern, regardless of its effects upon the flow of traffic). Responses such as the knee jerk and the eye blink in man are prime examples of open-loop behavior in which the basic response pattern, once initiated, cannot be altered to any significant degree. Adams, however, has cited evidence to show that feedback does play a role in open-loop behavior in lower animals, but is primarily confined to eliciting changes in the speed with which the stereotyped pattern is executed. Feedback cannot essentially alter the basic response pattern in open-loop behavior but can only augment the stimulus input and modify the rate and the intensity of the response. Feedback has also been shown to be a critical factor in initiating preprogramed species-specific responses such as song patterns in birds.

Closed-loop behavior, in contrast, is characterized by the continual modification and adjustment of the ongoing activity based upon information feedback from the response itself. A common example of a closed-loop system is the previously mentioned thermostatic regulation where changes in the environmental temperature affect the intensity of the activity of the heating or cooling machinery. The regulation of behavioral activities, however, is a far more complicated process.

Although feedback plays a critical role in the regulation and control of human behavior, complex activities such as motor skill acquisition cannot be described solely in closed-loop terms.

### Complexity and Interaction

Perhaps the respective roles of open-loop and closed-loop paradigms in motor learning can be more clearly understood by relating them to certain basic concepts of physical science. Just as atoms represent fundamental elements which combine in definite proportions to form more complex entities (molecules), the reflex is the fundamental element of all more complex movement patterns (subroutines). Viewing the reflex as the atom of behavior, one can see that individual reflexes function in an open-loop manner. The reflex, like the atom, has certain "built-in" properties which account for its particular behavior and, as in a chemical reaction, these properties can be altered through interaction with other reflexes. Just as the individual properties of sodium and chlorine are drastically altered in salt, or those of hydrogen and oxygen in water, the fundamental properties of individual reflexes can also be modified through the inhibitory effects of other reflexes which comprise a particular subroutine. Much of coordinated movement is in fact dependent upon the inhibition of reflex activities by higher centers in the nervous system.

The more complex the movement pattern, the more critical the role of information feedback in its acquisition and performance. Feedback conveys information concerning the need for motor adjustments and adaptations during the course of acquisition. These changes in the combination and patterning of the elements of a movement are in a way similar to variations in the proportions of different ingredients in a recipe to achieve a desired consistency. Feedback is also critical in the performance of a movement following its initial acquisition, for, just as the balance between the mutually attractive forces of the constituent atoms hold a molecule together, response-produced information feedback serves as the central factor unifying a complex movement pattern.

Complex behavior activities comprised of ordered patterns of subroutines and directed toward attaining a particular goal or purpose (as opposed to stereotyped reflexive responses) are classified as molar behavior. (See Chapter 2) Although comprised of a large number of elements, the unified properties of molar behavior far exceed the sum of the individual properties of each of its elements. Just as a house has properties that exceed those of the materials employed in its construction, molar behavior possesses properties unique to its particular level of organization. Skiing, swimming, dance, and gymnastics are readily recognized examples of molar behavior because of their unique patterns of organization. A complex motor activity is characterized by a precise pattern of temporal and spatial organization and, according to Gentile and Nacson (1976), any attempt to reduce such an ordered system to a detailed description of its components often results in a loss of the characteristics that define the system.

It is not the simple addition of the components of the activity, but rather the ordered regularity governing the interactions among these components, that distinguishes molar behavior. Molar behavior is the product of complex interactions and cannot be classified solely as either open-loop or closed-loop since the role of feedback in its execution varies with such factors as the timing of the movement and the level of conscious control exerted by the learner.

### Reference Mechanisms

Schmidt (1976a) hypothesizes a spatial-temporal pattern or motor program which, although highly complex, functions in an open-loop manner for a given duration before any adjustment based upon response-produced feedback can be effected. The minimum time required for such an adjustment is one reaction time, which can vary from approximately 200 msc. for visual and auditory information to about 110 msc. for proprioception. It appears that given the reaction time delay, all movements, regardless of their complexity, are initiated in an open-loop fashion.

Complex motor activity involves two fundamental processes, selection and initiation (open-loop functions), and regulation and control (closed-loop processes). Adams (1971) contends that the choice, direction, and extent of a movement constitute the major factors in the regulation and control of intrinsically-paced, voluntarily induced motor activity. However, the precise displacement of a limb segment requires a reference value related to previous movements which contain some trace of the preceding activity. Much information is essential in order to process the response-produced feedback concerning the momentary position of the involved body segment. Although the learner must possess some reference standard in order to process feedback information meaningfully, controversy exists concerning the respective roles of biological and environmental factors in the programing of these reference mechanisms. Adams argues that the strength of the reference mechanism increases as a positive function of the learner's growing experience of the proprioceptive, tactual, visual, and auditory feedback which emanate from each performance of a motor task. Although it is generally accepted that experience plays a critical role in strengthening and refining these mechanisms, there is disagreement concerning the role of environmental and hereditary factors in their initial programing.

Determinists argue that biological factors alone account for the quality of the reference centers. Behaviorists contend that environmental factors are central in their programing. Although biological factors play a role in the programing of reference mechanisms, they are primarily confined to the control of simple reflexive behavior and diminish in importance in the mediation of complex molar behavior which involves cognitive activity. The greater the complexity of the behavior and the more critical the role of cognition in its elicitation and control, the greater the role of experience and learning in the programing of the reference centers which regulate these complex behaviors.

*The Perceptual Trace.* Adams (1971) hypothesized two distinct reference mechanisms: the memory trace, critical in the initiation of voluntary movement; and the perceptual trace, which is central in the regulation and control of such movement. The perceptual trace is strengthened through the repetition of the movements occurring on each trial, but weakened as a consequence of forgetting. The transition from dependence upon verbal feedback during the initial stages of skill acquisition to proprioceptive feedback during the later stages may well lie in the state of the perceptual trace itself. Since the perceptual trace is weak during the early stages of learning, and reference values are not well established, the presentation of knowledge of results strengthens it by defining more sharply the correct response through reinforced practice. As proficiency develops, the reference mechanism is continually refined and the learner develops the capacity to process proprioceptive information. Until the perceptual trace is well established, however, the learner has no reference standard for the interpretation of the proprioceptive feedback from the response.

*The Memory Trace.* Adams argues the existence of a second factor, broader in scope than the perceptual trace, which selects and initiates complex patterns of behavior. This second factor, or memory trace, is believed to exert its function by translating verbalization and ideation into movement. It complements the perceptual trace, which functions as a reference mechanism by matching the actual feedback from a given response with the desired pattern elicited by the memory trace.

Schmidt (1975b) critically evaluates Adams' theoretical position and concludes that although it deals with learning and performance variables, and is well delimited in scope, clearly stated, and supported by empirical evidence, it is nonetheless characterized by a series of conspicuous shortcomings.

First, Adams' theory is predicated primarily upon data obtained from the study of slow, precise positioning movements. The application of these theoretical conclusions to the acquisition of gross motor skills, particularly when they must be executed under speeded conditions, is subject to question.

Second, Adams' theory implies that learning can continue in the absence of KR. Schmidt contends, however, that if the desired response is less than perfect on the first no-KR trial, the perceptual trace will be degraded as a consequence of the feedback from that response. Since the perceptual trace has been weakened, the succeeding response will be adversely affected and will, in turn, result in a further erosion of the perceptual trace. Schmidt concludes, therefore, that performance in the absence of KR can percipitate a chain of events which may result in the eventual total breakdown of the perceptual trace.

Third, Adams' theory fails to account for the learner's capacity to adapt and generalize a given response to a variety of situations. Since the probability of the occurrence of two identical stimulus situations is low, the learner would have to store a separate motor program to deal with every possible response contingency (an enormous number of programs), an alternative which, purely from the logistical standpoint, appears untenable.

Fourth, Adams fails to describe adequately the nature of the neurological mechanisms which govern the translation of proprioceptive feedback (information derived from the speed and position of the limb segments) into precise patterns of efferent discharge (information regulating the intensity and duration of muscular contraction).

Schmidt's criticism of Adams' work is amplified by Gentile and Nacson (1976), who contend that Adams' theory is fundamentally peripheral in nature since it views the learner as playing a basically passive role in the acquisition process. The authors argue that Adams views learning as a gradual incremental development of internal states affected only by external events with no regard for intrinsic organizational processes. Gentile and Nacson object to Adams' assumption regarding movement-produced feedback as the central factor in the mediation of motor behavior since this position implies that learning is a product of random external events rather than a result of organized intrinsic processes. In summary, the authors contend that Adams' theoretical positions are based upon reductionist concepts which fail to account adequately for the transformational processes or relational rules which link the level of information feedback to the higher level functions of evaluation and correction.

### Knowledge of Results

Knowledge of results is a form of augmented feedback, verbal in nature and externally manipulated at the discretion of the teacher or experimenter. Adams (1978) writes that KR is a form of extrinsic terminal feedback which reinforces goal-directed acts (molar behavior) as opposed to isolated movements (molecular behavior). He contends that KR is critical during the initial stages of acquisition in which the standards of correctness for processing the stimulus input are unknown to the learner. The KR administrator (the teacher or coach), who is familiar with these standards, provides verbal information which enables the learner to reduce the degree of discrepancy (error message) between the response desired and the one attained. Since the learner ultimately internalizes this information, the need for KR is greatly diminished as learning progresses. Bilodeau (1966) writes that the term "knowledge of results" pertains only to the amount of information provided by the experimenter and is separate and independent of any knowledge or perceptions the student receives through the actual performance of the task itself.

Bourne (1966) observes that a high level of information feedback is often an intrinsic factor in many motor skills since the subject can often be aware of the consequences of his response in the absence of any extrinsic KR. Bowling and foul shots in basketball are prime examples of activities in which the consequences of the response provide the subject with a level of KR sufficiently accurate to enable him to modify or sustain that response. Since research dealing with the role of KR in motor learning is concerned with the effects of experimenter-controlled information feedback, the criterion tasks employed in such studies must provide relatively little inherent feedback.

Studies concerned with the effects of KR upon the acquisition of motor skills, in addition to constraining the selection of the criterion task, entail depriving the subject of some form of sensory feedback and supplanting it with extrinsic verbal information. Although it is visual feedback which is most frequently withheld, studies have been also designed which seek to deprive subjects of proprioceptive feedback. Visual feedback can effectively be eliminated by the use of a blindfold, but sensory deprivation of proprioceptive feedback entails physical compression of the involved limb segment's nerves, a technique of questionable effectiveness.

Regardless of the nature of the sensory feedback withheld, all studies concerned with the role of knowledge of results in motor learning employ a basic experimental design. While all subjects are deprived of some form of sensory feedback, half are provided with a knowledge of the results of their actions and the remaining half receive no such information. The nature of the verbal information provided concerning the accuracy of the learner's response may be dichotomous (as in the children's game of "hot and cold") and confined to such qualitative statements as "yes" or "no," "good" or "poor," "true" or "false," "right" or "wrong," and "pass" or "fail," or may be instead a precise quantitative statement of performance measured along some previously defined response continuum.

Studies of the latter type provide the subject with information concerning the magnitude and/or direction of the error, such as "five degrees too far to the left." In summarizing the findings of studies employing quantitative knowledge of results, Schmidt (1975a) observed that providing subjects with knowledge of the direction of their error yielded performance superior to the results obtained when subjects were provided with information concerning only the magnitude of the error. The best results, however, were achieved when information pertaining to the magnitude and the direction of the error was provided.

Reeve and Magill (1981) observed that although the typical KR statement may convey information concerning the direction and the magnitude of error, it is the former information which proves most critical during the initial acquisition of a linear positioning task. As proficiency develops, subjects are able to make increased use of KR dealing with magnitude of error even though they are given no prior information concerning the nature of the units employed to measure distance. In order for KR to serve as an external reference standard, the learner must first develop an understanding of the information contained therein. The authors contend that the learner's capacity to process certain forms of KR is a result of the repeated pairing (contiguous association) of the sensory consequences of a response (the intrinsic feedback) with the KR statement itself. Through this paired association, the learner develops some form of internal labeling system or reference mechanism for processing the extrinsic information (the KR).

Newell (1976) writes that KR which provides the subject with precise quantitative information yields performance superior to that obtained if either imprecise or qualitative KR is given. This contention is substantiated in part by the findings of Shapiro (1977), who observed that preschool children who received highly precise KR made fewer errors on a linear positioning task than those who received less precise KR. Predicated upon these findings, it is logical to conclude that, in general, the more specific the KR, the higher the level of performance and the more rapid the improvement.

This is not absolutely true, however, since the optimum level of KR specificity is relative to such factors as the age and ability level of the learner and the complexity of the task. Finally, there is no absolute optimum value of KR specificity which will ensure the most efficient learning in every situation. An experienced tennis instructor will more likely provide instructions and corrections which are complicated and precise in nature to an adult pupil than to a child, since the adult possesses a greater capacity to process such KR.

### Delay of KR

Knowledge of results need not be presented immediately after every single trial to be effective. Schmidt (1975a) defines the time between a given response and its succeeding response as the interresponse interval, which is itself divisible into two components. The time between the response and the knowledge of results, termed the KR delay, is the first. The second is termed the post-KR delay and is comprised of the interval between the KR and the succeeding response. It appears logical that there are different processes taking place during the KR delay and the post-KR delay intervals because the subject most likely stores information about the previous response while awaiting the KR, and alters and adjusts his actions in accordance with the information received following the KR.

Although delay of reinforcement proves detrimental to learning in studies involving animals, delay of KR apparently has no adverse effect upon human learning. This is evidenced by the findings of studies which reveal that the KR delay interval can be varied from a matter of seconds up to one week with no apparent consequences upon the acquisition of criterion measures. If, however, the KR is delayed for more than one response interval, i.e., there are a number of intervening trials between the initial response and the KR for that particular response, there is a great deal of interference with the learning of the task. Predicated upon these observations, the major difference between knowledge of results and reinforcement appears to be the informational properties of KR, not its properties of reward.

Newell (1976) writes that the emphasis of current research concerning the effects of KR upon motor learning has shifted from a position which viewed KR primarily in terms of its properties of reinforcement to one which views it in terms of its informational value. As a consequence of this altered perspective, there has been an accompanying change in the focus of attention from the KR delay period to the post-KR interval. The processing of the KR and the resultant formulation of the appropriate strategies for executing the succeeding response are believed to occur in this later phase of the intertrial interval. Newell contends that the post-KR interval must be sustained for some minimal period in order for KR to be processed effectively, and the temporal duration of this period will vary directly with the complexity of the task and the precision of the KR.

Despite the currently prevailing position which views the role of KR in learning as primarily informational, a number of current investigations dealing with the effects of the length of the post-KR interval on acquisition have failed to substantiate this contention. Boucher (1974) observed no differences in acquisition rate between subjects receiving post-KR intervals of three seconds and ten seconds. Magill (1973) found no differences in acquisition rate between groups receiving post-KR periods of two seconds and thirty seconds. Newell contends that these findings are the result of the highly simplistic nature of the criterion tasks employed since the KR-processing time for these activities was most probably less than the shortest post-KR delay period employed in either study.

Magill (1977) provided further evidence against the position that KR is primarily informational in nature when he observed that neither varying the length of the post-KR interval nor introducing an interfering activity during the interval affected the rate of acquisition of a serial positioning task. He contends, however, that this discrepancy between theoretical prediction and empirical observation may be due to the simplicity of criterion tasks which are characteristically employed in KR delay studies. Magill argues, therefore, that theoretical predictions which concern the effects of manipulating the post-KR interval and which are based upon empirical data derived from studies employing such simplistic criterion tasks may well be inappropriate to studies dealing with the acquisition of complex motor skills.

Magill views the acquisition of simple tasks as a function of short-term memory and the learning of complex tasks as a function of long-term memory. Although the role of KR information properties may be uncertain in the short-term memory processes which underlie the acquisition of simple tasks, the information conveyed by the KR becomes more critical as the complexity of the task increases and the learning process comes to involve long-term memory functions. This conclusion appears logically sound; the greater the complexity of the task, the greater the role of cognitive activity in acquisition and recall.

The arguments favoring the informational properties of knowledge of results are substantiated by Adams (1971), who argues that motor learning is best viewed as a problem-solving activity in which the learner can discover the required movement only through the KR he receives. Adams contends that a learner may not always employ the KR in a direct fashion, but may instead use it to form strategies and hypotheses concerning the solution of the motor problem. In the case of human learning, the KR may only be a starting point, however, since it is the cognitive activity elicited by the information feedback rather than the feedback itself which directly influences the motor behavior.

The acquisition of complex motor skills is contingent upon a great deal of interaction between verbal and motor systems. Cognitive factors tend to play a more critical role during the initial phase of motor skill acquisition but diminish in importance during the course of learning due to a decreased dependence upon verbal information as proficiency develops. Although Adams' findings are generally accepted, controversy exists concerning the respective roles of proprioceptive information and central neurological control mechanisms in the acquisition of motor skills. Opinion is divided between theorists who contend that peripheral feedback is central in skill acquisition and those who argue that motor learning is the result of preprogramed, central neurological processes which are capable of exerting their control functions in the absence of feedback.

Schendel and Newell (1976) have reviewed the arguments for both positions and conclude that although the belief that the learner actively processes feedback information at a cognitive level holds much intuitive appeal, experiments dealing with the problem have yielded conflicting results. Research findings generally reveal that there is an optimum post-KR interval for the acquisition of a given activity. Increasing this interval beyond its optimum point will have no incremental effect upon acquisition, but decreasing its temporal duration will exert a pronounced decremental effect. The critical factor in determining the optimum length of the post-KR interval is the complexity of the criterion task.

Viewed within the context of information theory, learning a complex task requires the subject to process a greater amount of information than learning a simple task. If the amount of information is increased while the length of the post-KR interval remains the same, a decremental effect results. Just as the increased complexity of a task results in more information to be processed, so, too, does the increased precision of the KR itself. As the precision of KR is increased, performance diminishes unless there is a corresponding increase in the length of the post-KR interval. Rogers (1974) writes that exceptionally precise KR exerts a detrimental effect because it presents the subject with an excessive amount of information to be processed in the time available. If the precision of the KR is held constant and the post-KR interval is shortened, performance is also adversely affected since the subject has less time in which to process the information.

Gallagher and Thomas (1980) observed that when children were given increased KR-processing time, their performance on a ballistic linear positioning task improved to a point not significantly different from that of adults. There is an optimal length for the post-KR interval which is dependent upon the complexity of the task and the precision of the information feedback obtained.

Adams summarizes the findings of research dealing with the effects of knowledge of results on the acquisition of motor skills in a series of tentative conclusions:

1. The improvement of performance in motor learning is dependent upon KR, and the rate of such improvement is dependent upon the precision of the KR.
2. The initial stages of motor learning are under verbal-cognitive control, i.e., subjects consciously mediate their movements and tend to verbalize self-corrections.
3. Delay of KR has little or no effect upon acquisition, provided the interresponse interval is held constant. The strength of the perceptual trace is dependent upon the length of the interresponse interval rather than the locus of the KR within this interval. If the interresponse interval is excessively long, the perceptual trace is weakened and the quality of the response declines. The only constraint placed upon the positioning of the KR within the interresponse interval is that the learner have sufficient time for processing the information.
4. Increasing the post-KR delay will improve performance level, provided such a delay falls within prescribed limits, since the learner requires time to process information.
5. The interpolation of verbal and/or motor activities in either the KR or post-KR delay interval does not appear to influence acquisition adversely as long as KR is present.

When knowledge of results is deliberately withdrawn or withheld, the following consequences have been observed:

1. Although the withdrawal of KR always produces deterioration of performance when level of training is low or moderate, learning can continue in the absence of KR, provided a relatively high degree of proficiency had been attained prior to its withdrawal.
2. If KR is delayed and the subject rests during this interval, the effects of KR withdrawal upon performance are the same as those obtained when immediate KR has been employed and then withdrawn.
3. When KR is delayed in acquisition and the subject engages in deliberate verbal or motor activity during the delay interval, the negative effects of KR withdrawal upon performance are greater than

those obtained when the subject remains at rest during the KR interval.

4. Any activity in the post-KR interval during acquisition worsens performance when KR is withdrawn.

Much of the current information dealing with the effects of knowledge of results upon motor learning is derived from experimental studies which employ criterion tasks of low complexity. The primary purpose of these studies has been concerned with establishing the effects of knowledge of results as a factor in and of itself, uncomplicated by the learner's ability to perform the task. The successful execution of the criterion activity must therefore be heavily dependent upon the immediately preceding KR rather than upon the ability, practice, learning, or skill of the subject.

Bilodeau and Jones (1970) write that such tasks as lever positioning or line drawing are selected precisely because of their uncomplex nature, which makes them well suited to KR studies. Even though there is a tendency to dismiss the findings of such studies as mere artifacts, the principles which govern the effects of KR upon simple tasks are also applicable in the case of complex, goal-directed activities.

Knowledge of results is particularly important during the initial acquisition of a skill, since practice in the absence of KR results in a mere repetition of the same errors and the ultimate acquisition of an incorrect response. This occurrence is particularly evident in the case of the "self-taught" performer who learns a response which partially fulfills the objective or goal of the movement but is grossly inefficient and often largely ineffective. The self-taught bowler who employs an improper approach and delivery but occasionally manages to succeed at knocking down some pins, or the self-taught swimmer who, by wildly kicking and flailing, is able to negotiate a minimal distance after expending an excessive amount of energy, are examples of the deleterious effects of practice which is not reinforced by knowledge of results.

There are several research findings concerning the effects of KR on motor learning which are particularly applicable to the teaching of complex, goal-directed, gross motor activities. The first of these pertains to the point at which KR should be introduced into the learning situation. Although it is important at all levels of learning, KR exerts its most important effects during the initial stages of acquisition when proficiency levels are low. At this point the learner has no basis for distinguishing a correct response from an incorrect one. Unless practice is reinforced by KR, it is equally probable that an incorrect response pattern will ultimately be acquired.

The second factor pertains to the interval between the response and the KR. While KR can be effective even if it is temporally delayed (within limits), its effects are greatly reduced if a second (competing) activity is introduced in the pre-KR interval (the time intervening between the initial response and the KR). In order to maximize the effectiveness of KR, it must be presented directly (although not necessarily immediately) following the response for which it is intende. intended. A teacher who wishes to provide a student with a knowledge of the results of his actions upon a particular trial must do so before the student executes another attempt. If the teacher fails to provide the KR at the right moment, its effectiveness is lost.

The third factor pertains to the precision of the KR itself. Imprecise KR will exert a minimal effect upon performance, but KR that is overly precise will prove equally ineffective. The precision of the KR must be adapted to the capacity of the learner; an adult can process more precise KR than a child. The KR must convey information precise enough to allow the learner to effect the appropriate response corrections but not so precise that it exceeds his information-processing capacity.

The fourth factor pertains to the duration of the interval following the KR. Since there must be sufficient time for the KR to be processed, the optimum length of this interval will vary with the proficiency of the learner and with the precision of the KR itself. During the initial stages of acquisition, there are wide fluctuations in the pattern of performance, and the learner must process large amounts of KR in order to effect the adjustments which will ultimately result in reducing the discrepancy between the response desired and the one actually obtained. These wide fluctuations in performance will diminish and KR-processing time will decrease as proficiency is developed. As the amount of KR required decreases, its precision must increase since the response pattern becomes more refined.

One of the major characteristics of the learning process itself pertains to the differences in the nature of the KR required during the early and late stages of skill acquisition. Since the learner must process large amounts of KR during the initial phase of acquisition, the post-KR period must be sufficiently lengthy to allow for the processing of great amounts of information. Although the amount of KR diminishes as proficiency is increased, the post-KR interval must still be long enough to allow for the processing of the more precise KR which is required in the later stages of learning.

*References*

Adams, J.A. "A Closed-Loop Theory of Motor Learning." *Journal of Motor Behavior, 3* (1971), 111–149.

_____. "Issues for a Closed-Loop Theory of Motor Learning." *In* G.E. Stelmach (ed.), *Motor Control Issues and Trends*. New York: Academic Press, 1976.

_____. "Theoretical Issues for Knowledge of Results." *In* G.E.Stelmach (ed.), *Information Processing in Motor Control and Learning*. New York: Academic Press, 1978.

Bilodeau, I.M. "Information Feedback." *In* E.A. Bilodeau (ed.), *Acquisition of Skill*. New York: Academic Press, 1966.

_____and M.B. Jones. "Information Feedback in Positioning: Problems and Progress." *In* L.E. Smith (ed.), *Psychology of Motor Learning*. Chicago: The Athletic Institute, 1970.

Boucher, J.C. "Higher Processes in Motor Learning." *Journal of Motor Behavior, 6* (1974), 131–137.

Bourne, L.E. "Information Feedback: Comments on Professor I.M. Bilodeau's Paper." *In* E.A. Bilodeau (ed.), *Acquisition of Skill*. New York: Academic Press, 1966.

Fleishman, E.A. "Individual Differences and Motor Learning." *In* R.M. Gagné (ed.), *Learning and Individual Differences*. Columbus, Ohio: Merrill, 1967.

Gallagher, J.D. and J.R. Thomas. "Effects of Varying Post-KR Intervals Upon Children's Motor Performance." *Journal of Motor Behavior, 12* (1980), 41–56.

Gentile, A.M. and J. Nacson. "Organizational Processes in Motor Control." *In* J. Keogh and R.S. Hutton (eds.), *Exercise and Sport Science Reviews*. Santa Barbara, Cal.: Journal Publishing Affiliates, 1976.

Magill, R.A. "The Post-KR Interval: Time and Activity Effects and the Relationship of Motor Short-Term Memory Theory." *Journal of Motor Behavior, 5* (1973), 49–56.

_____. "The Processing of Knowledge of Results Information for a Serial-Motor Task." *Journal of Motor Behavior, 9* (1977), 113–118.

Newell, K.M. "Knowledge of Results and Motor Learning." *In* J. Keogh and R.S. Hutton (eds.), *Exercise and Sport Science Reviews*. Santa Barbara, Cal.: Journal Publishing Affiliates, 1976.

Reeve, T.G. and R.A. Magill. "The Role of the Components of Knowledge of Results Information in Error Correction." *Research Quarterly for Exercise and Sport, 52* (1981), 80–85.

Robb, M. *Dynamics of Motor Skill Acquisition*. Englewood Cliffs, NJ: Prentice-Hall, 1972.

Rogers, C.A. "Feedback Precision and Postfeedback Interval Duration." *Journal of Experimental Psychology, 102* (1974), 604–608.

Schendel, J.D. and K.M. Newell. "On Processing the Information from

Knowledge of Results." *Journal of Motor Behavior, 8* (1976), 251–255.

Schmidt, R.A. *Motor Skills.* New York: Harper and Row, 1975a.

————. "A Schema Theory of Discrete Motor Skill Learning." *Psychological Review, 85* (1975b), 225–260.

————. "Control Processes in Motor Skills." *In* J. Keogh and R.S. Hutton (eds.), *Exercise and Sport Science Reviews.* Santa Barbara, Cal.: Journal Publishing Affiliates, 1976a.

————. "The Schema as a Solution to Some Persistent Problems in Motor Learning Theory." *In* G.E.Stelmach (ed.), *Motor Control Issues and Trends.* New York: Academic Press, 1976b.

Shapiro, D.C. "Knowledge of Results and Motor Learning in Preschool Children." *Research Quarterly, 48* (1977), 154–158.

Smith, K.U. and G. "Feedback Mechanism of Athletic Skill." *In* L.E. Smith (ed.), *Psychology of Motor Learning.* Chicago: The Athletic Institute, 1970.

Wiener, N. *Cybernetics.* New York: John Wiley, 1948.

# CHAPTER 9

# Motor Retention and Information-Processing Models of Motor Control

IN ADDITION TO the intensive research on the effects of post-KR interval length upon learning, attention has been focused on the effects produced when various types of verbal and motor activities are interpolated into this interval. Theorists favoring a cognitive viewpoint hold that since the learner must actively process and act upon the knowledge of results, the interpolation of any activities within the post-KR interval will exert a decremental effect upon acquisition. Although the study of motor retention is confounded by a number of specific, critical, methodological problems, the major theoretical issues which prevail in this area of research are rooted in verbal learning. Melton (1970) writes that a fundamental controversy pertains to the nature of the processes which account for short-term memory (STM)* and long-term memory (LTM).* Theorists who view memory as a continuum contend that STM and LTM are linked by an unbroken transition process. Researchers who view the processes of memory as discrete components argue that they represent two distinct mechanisms with wholly different characteristics.

## Motor Retention

In general, proponents of the continuum theory of memory view forgetting as a consequence of interference which may be the result of proactive inhibition or retroactive inhibition. Advocates of the discrete nature of STM and LTM relate forgetting to the spontaneous decay of the memory trace over time. Those theorists who believe that STM and LTM are components of the same process argue that the degree of interference is directly related to the degree of similarity between the criterion activity, or "to-be-remembered unit" (TBRU), and a preceding or an interpolated task. When interference results from prior exposure to a similar task, it is called proactive, and when it results from the interpolation of a similar task, it is called retroactive.

---

*STM involves the storage of information for periods of thirty seconds or less; LTM, for periods greater than thirty seconds.

The views of Broadbent (1970) are an exception to this theoretical position. He advocates a two-factor theory of memory, but agrees that the control factor in all forms of forgetting is interference. In the case of STM, any form of interference is believed to result in a loss of retention. The degree of interference with LTM processes is believed to be in direct ratio to the degree of similarity between the criterion task and the competing activity. The greater the similarity (e.g., the forehand in tennis and badminton), the greater the interference and consequent forgetting. Conversely, the greater the dissimilarity between the two activities, the less the forgetting and the greater the retention.

Tulving (1970) writes that recent experimental evidence tends to support the position that STM and LTM represent discrete mechanisms which exert independent functions. This departure from the traditional view of memory as a continuum is based upon findings which reveal that a number of variables produce different effects upon recall at different retention intervals. Tulving cites three events which comprise an act of memory: the input of information into the store, the storage of information or maintenance of the store, and the retrieval of information from the store. Although theorists are concerned with how STM and LTM differ in terms of all three of these functions, the major distinction appears to be the differences in the storage processes peculiar to the two forms of memory.

The STM store is thought to possess a strictly limited capacity. All incoming information is either continually replaced by subsequent input or, unless actively rehearsed, spontaneously decays over time. Broadbent (1970) writes that a common example of the limitations of short-term memory is an individual trying to retain a phone number which has been presented verbally. He must write down the number immediately after learning it or continually repeat the number verbally (active rehearsal) until the call is completed. If the individual cannot write down the number and is wholly dependent upon active rehearsal for its retention, anything blocking this rehearsal process (e.g., a third party asking the caller a question before he begins to dial) will cause all or part of the information retained in the short-term memory store to be lost.

In contrast, the long-term memory store is believed to have a much greater capacity for holding information, all of which it selectively receives from the short-term store. Tulving (1970) argues that the major disinction between STM and LTM is differences in the mechanisms which retrieve information from the memory store rather than any differences between the actual memory stores themselves. This argument is based upon the fact that recall performance depends not only upon the availability of information in the store (i.e., the amount retained), but upon the accessibility of the information as well.

Tulving theorizes that the actual accessibility of information stored in memory is a function of the availability of specific stimuli or retrieval cues which have been previously associated with the criterion response and can be utilized by the learner at the time of recall. The nature of these retrieval cues is believed to be determined by coding processes which may entail the qualitative (verbal) or quantitative (numerical) labeling of information pertaining to the recall of the criterion response. These cues, or ancillary information, are stored along with the criterion response following initial acquisition and facilitate the recall of the to-be-remembered unit. Since the retrieval cues are always less complex in nature than the TBRU, they are more accessible and thus facilitate the recall of the TBRU. The effectiveness of a retrieval cue relies entirely upon the strength of its association with the criterion response.

Quantitative coding may require a numerical designation of each individual element in a coordinated sequence of behavior, particularly when the sequencing calls for precise temporal integration. A gymnast, for example, might recall the individual moves in his routine through the application of a quantitative coding system in which each move is labeled in terms of its ordinal sequence and temporal duration. Qualitative coding or verbal labeling may consist of an alphabetical designation, such as the first letter in the name of the TBRU, some sound associated with this name, or the name itself. The extent to which verbal labels contribute to the recall of motor skills, however, is not yet clearly understood. Tulving writes that the retention of verbal information appears to involve different retrieval cues for STM and LTM: short-term memory involves quantitative temporal cues; the long-term memory store is dependent upon more qualitative semantic cues.

*Interference and Spontaneous Decay* There are also differences in the nature of the activities which interfere with the processes of LTM and STM. Broadbent (1970) writes that information retained in short-term memory is most prone to interference from the introduction of competing material which manifests a high degree of physical similarity to the original material retained in the store. The more the competing response sounds or feels like the TBRU, the greater the resultant interference. In the case of long-term memory, interference results from the degree of similarity between the meaning or concept underlying the TBRU and those concepts which underlie the competing material, i.e., from conceptual similarity rather than physical resemblance. Common examples of conceptual interference with LTM store are a student employing an incorrect formula on an algebra exam because the correct formula and the one selected are so similar, or a student in a comparative literature class who cannot remember which quotes are cited from which works of the author under study.

Much current research is rooted in the theoretical controversies concerning the nature and function of STM and LTM. Schendel and Newell (1976), after reviewing the literature, write that interpolated kinesthetic activities apparently do not interfere with information processing during the post-KR interval since activities of this type do not seem to interfere with central processing operations. The authors conclude that any interference resulting from the interpolation of a kinesthetic activity will be confined to those activities which place demands primarily upon the learner's capacities for memory and recall. In other words, the mere performance of an interpolated kinesthetic activity during the post-KR interval exerts no apparent decremental effect upon acquisition unless this act itself entails some form of cognitive activity.

Schendel and Newell contend that a major factor which determines the extent of the interference caused by the interpolation of an activity in the post-KR interval is the pacing of that activity. They believe that the learning of activities which are intrinsically-paced is less prone to interference from the interpolation of an alternative activity during the post-KR delay interval than the learning of extrinsically (experimenter) paced activities. In the former, the subject has a greater opportunity to process the information at a rate which is most beneficial to him. In the case of intrinsically-paced tasks, for example, the processing of KR may not only be confined to the post-KR interval, but may occur as the subject is actually performing the task. Schendel and Newell contend that an intrinsically-paced task provides the learner with an opportunity to process KR covertly while actively performing the task.

Laabs (1976) studied the relationship between the taxonomy of the interpolated activity and the degree of interference with the learning of the criterion task. Two forms of interference, capacity and structural, were distinguished. Capacity interference results from the interpolation of an activity which competes with the criterion task for the available central processing time allotted for the acquisition of both. The greater the demands of the interpolated activity upon the central processing mechanism, the greater the resultant capacity interference. An interpolated movement which has to be committed to long-term memory will result in capacity interference. Structural interference, on the other hand, is a form of negative transfer in which the interpolated activity retroactively inhibits the acquisition of the criterion task. In this case, the interpolated activity is relegated to the short-term memory store and no demand is made upon central processing capacity. The degree of structural interference is a function of the similarity between the criterion task and the interpolated task; it is zero when the two tasks are identical and maximal when they are highly similar.

Laabs writes that tasks which require the subject to process kinesthetic information about the end location of a movement require central processing operations. When activities of this nature are interpolated in the post-KR interval, capacity interference results and has a decremental effect upon the acquisition of the criterion task. When the interpolated activity is remembering information about the distance of the movement, however, only short-term processes appear to be involved and interference is confined to the structural type.

Adams and Dijkstra (1966) caution that apparent similarities observed between verbal short-term memory and motor short-term memory may be due to a substantial verbal component embodied in the criterion motor task used for a particular study. Since it is widely acknowledged that implicit verbal responses can facilitate motor behavior under certain task conditions, subjects could possibly employ a covert verbal label to help define the motor response. (A diver might think the word "tuck" before executing a backward dive in tuck position.) An erroneous motor response could then be attributed to processes associated with verbal learning, forgetting processes which, in turn, result in the recall of a wrong verbal label.

The authors argue that, as in the case of verbal learning, the motor-memory trace becomes increasingly stable as it proceeds from short-term to long-term memory store and that reinforcement strengthens the trace just as time weakens it. However, it was observed that as the post-KR interval increased, forgetting increased. Since this interval was not filled by any competing activity, the subject had an optimal opportunity to rehearse the motor response actively and should, therefore, have manifested an increment in performance directly proportional to the duration of the post-KR interval. The observed results conflicted with this position—performance declined as the length of the interval increased. Adams and Dijkstra contend that the primary source of interference with the motor-memory trace results from the decay of the memory trace over time, not from proactive or retroactive inhibitory effects.

Stelmach and Wilson (1970) write that the degree to which motor memory is dependent upon central information-processing (channel) capacity is not clearly understood. Motor retention apparently requires less conscious rehearsal than the retention of verbal information. In an investigation of the relationship between task definition and motor retention, Stelmach, Kelso, and McCullagh (1976) observed that performance upon constrained or experimenter-paced tasks was far more prone to spontaneous decay following an unfilled retention interval of fifteen seconds than performance upon preselected or subject-defined tasks. The authors report that the subject's superior retention of the preselected task is due to the possession of precise information concerning the extent and the terminal location of the movement prior to its execution. This information is centrally processed and readily retrievable following the retention interval. In a constrained task, however, the subject has no prior knowledge of the extent of the movement and simply proceeds until directed to stop. Performance is dependent upon the continuous monitoring of peripheral feedback information, but there is no central model with which the feedback can be compared. As a consequence, the subject is unable to retain the information, and performance decays following an unfilled retention interval.

Marteniuk (1976) argues that the superior retention of unconstrained, subject-defined movements results from the ability to encode in the short-term memory story a nonverbal image, or spatial map, detailing the characteristics of the criterion response. Subjects performing experimenter-defined or constrained tasks are unable to formulate an equally accurate image of the task and, hence, demonstrate poorer retention. Regardless of the nature of the criterion task, the spatial image is believed to decay spontaneously over a period of twenty seconds unless it is integrated with information from other sensory modalities, such as vision and audition. Marteniuk theorizes that the long-term retention of an internal representation of a physical movement (long-term motor memory) is critically dependent upon the integration of proprioceptive and visual information.

The arguments raised by the findings of Adams and Dijkstra and Stelmach et al. are part of the broader question concerning the respective roles of interference and memory trace decay in retention and forgetting. Proponents of interference theory view forgetting as the consequence of a previously acquired response trace spontaneously reappearing and interfering with the current acquisition of the criterion response (negative transfer or structural interference). Advocates of the trace decay theory contend that forgetting can occur in the absence of any interference effects, either capacity or structural, because the memory trace will decay as a function of time alone. Gentile and Nacson (1976) write that the major problem in resolving this question is the difficulty of subjecting the theoretical positions to experimental tests. A test of the decay theory would require that the time factor be manipulated independently of the execution of the interpolated activity. The very nature of the criterion tasks employed in these retention studies (i.e., positioning tasks), however, requires an interpolated activity in order to reproduce the original task.

Gentile and Nacson are critical on theoretical as well as methodological grounds of current research upon the retention of motor skills. They contend that contemporary theories of motor retention simplistically view the learner as a passive receiver and transmitter of information, relegated to performing a static intermediary function between stimulus and response. They argue that these theories are inadequate because they fail to deal with the dynamic central processes governing the transformation of information and the organization and direction of the learner's activities before and during the retention interval. Gentile and Nacson conclude that much of the conflicting data in this area is attributable to the lack of a unifying body of theory and to the wide variations in such methodological considerations as type of interference, length of the retention interval, number of repetitions, and method of presentation.

_Measures of Motor Retention._ Many variables—task taxonomy, method of presentation, length of the post-KR interval, retention, and the nature of the interpolated activity, as well as the specific method employed to measure performance upon the task—affect research in this area. Roy (1976) writes that there are four performance measures which have been consistently employed to assess performance in the area of motor retention: absolute error (AE), constant error (CE), variable error (VE), and total variability (E).

AE measures the degree of deviation of a response without regard for sign or direction (absolute value); CE measures the degree of deviation of a response in terms of the magnitude and the direction of the error (algebraic value). When computing AE, the absolute value of each error is averaged over a number of trials. Assume that the criterion task required the learner to move a lever a distance of six inches. On the first trial, the subject moves the lever only five inches, on the second trial seven inches, on the third trial eight inches, and on each of the fourth and fifth trials, five inches. The subject was one inch short (- 1) of the goal on the first trial, two inches long (+2) on the second, three inches the long (+3) on the third, and one inch short (–1) on both the fourth and fifth trials. Since AE is computed upon the absolute error value of each trial, the subject's error in this case would be equal to $\frac{1 + 2 + 3 + 1 + 1}{5} = \frac{8}{5} = 1.6$. If, however, given the same data, the researcher had decided to employ CE, which is computed by averaging the algebraic sum of the individual error values, the subject's error score would be $\frac{1+2+3-1-1}{5} = \frac{2}{5} = .40.$ Clearly, differences in the error measure employed can drastically influence the findings of a study. Although AE and CE have been widely employed as criterion measures in studies dealing with motor retention and knowledge of results, both methods have conspicuous shortcomings. AE completely disregards the direction of the error, a factor which can be significant in and of itself. CE, predicated upon the algebraic sum of the individual response errors, often results in an unrealistically low error measure.

Due to a dissatisfaction with both AE and CE, the third measure, variable error, has been developed. Although the computation of VE requires greater mathematical sophistication than the others, VE preserves the algebraic integrity of each individual deviation without the resultant unrealistically low estimate of the error value. According to Schmidt (1975b), VE is actually the standard deviation of a subject's performance around his CE and is derived by the formula

$$VE = \sqrt{\sum \frac{(X_t - CE)^2}{n}}$$

where $X_t$ stands for the error score on a given trial and CE is the average error. By subtracting the CE from each trial, one can observe if performance on that trial is above or below the average, and thereby the information pertaining to the direction of the error is preserved. Square these differences and all minus signs become positive, yielding a sum that is truly representative of the range of error. By taking the square root of the expression, the research obtains an error value in original score terms which reflects deviations from the average without the loss of directional properties. The final measure, E or total variability, was introduced by Henry (1974) and is expressed by the formula $E = \sqrt{CE^2 + VE^2}$ .E represents the total variability of a subject's scores around a target.

Roy (1976) writes that despite controversy over the dependent measure to be employed in a given circumstance, there has been no consistent use of any of these measures. Theorists favoring a behavioristic view of motor retention tend to employ either AE or E as the measure of criterion performance; theorists favoring an information-processing view tend to employ either CE or VE. It is conceivable that the lack of consistency among the dependent measures employed in various studies dealing with motor retention constitutes a major factor contributing to the apparent disagreement among the findings of these studies.

## Motor Control

Although research on the retention and recall of motor skill is often complicated by methodological inconsistencies, findings in this area have nonetheless considerably advanced the understanding of the basis of motor control. Since the control of complex movement patterns depends upon the capacity to effect the appropriate behavioral adjustments in response to changes in the environmental input, the learner must possess some reference standard for evaluating information feedback in order to make these adjustments. Participation in ball sports, for example, not only requires the learner to make continual adaptation to changes in the speed and direction of the ball, but also involves his capacity to adjust to fluctuations in atmospheric and surface conditions (e.g., a shift in the wind or rocks or holes on the field).

The degree to which a reference mechanism or standard contributes to the processing of feedback information is dependent upon the quality and precision of its initial programing. The processes of motor retention and recall are basic elements in the programing of the reference mechanisms. Evaluation of ongoing behavior is dependent upon the retention and recall of information pertaining to the nature of the desired response. While most theorists agree upon the central role played by such mechanisms in the regulation and control of movement, there is considerable disagreement over the place of extrinsic and intrinsic feedback in the motor control process.

*Open- and Closed-Loop Models.* The respective roles of central and peripheral mechanisms in the processing of information feedback are matter for controversy. The classical closed-loop paradigm of motor control proposed by Sherrington envisions the learner as making continual adjustments in response to proprioceptive feedback from the periphery. Jones (1974a) contends that the peripheral feedback hypothesis is inadequate because the time required to process such information virtually precludes the possibility of controlled movements under highly speeded conditions. Schmidt (1975a) writes that although there is no conclusive experimental evidence to demonstrate that movement can occur in the absence of feedback, feedback-processing time requires approximately 200 msc. The fact that an individual is capable of eliciting complex speeded motor responses which exceed this information-processing capacity, however, is taken as indirect evidence supporting the concept of a central motor regulatory mechanism.

Proponents of theories advocating the primacy of central control in motor learning argue that the learner possesses a set of stored commands which are structured prior to the onset of the activity and which effect the entire movement sequence uninfluenced by peripheral feedback. Jones (1974b) hypothesizes a central regulatory mechanism or motor program, which he calls the CME, that monitors and retains efferent signals to the muscles. He contends that the CME accounts for an individual's capacity to retain a movement in the absence of feedback or instructional cues for an interval of up to fifteen seconds.

The arguments of Schmidt and Jones about the open-loop nature of motor control are substantiated by the findings of Newell (1976b), who observed that the learning of a rapid positioning movement was not adversely affected when practiced over a series of no-KR trials. Newell writes that the opportunity for evaluating feedback for response error detection during the course of the movement is denied when an activity is highly speeded. Due to limitations in information-processing rate and factors of reaction time latency, the accuracy of a rapid movement can be evaluated only after the movement has been completed. The feedback obtained from the outcome of the preceding response can then be employed to adjust response selection on the following trial. Newell contends that the central response-recognition mechanism is developed as a consequence of practice which is initially reinforced by KR. This recognition mechanism is believed to be programed with feedback information from preceding trials, enabling the learner to produce a correct response on any given trial in the absence of KR.

Jones (1974a) writes that physiologists have resorted traditionally to two distinct theories of motor control, both of which rest upon the assumption that the efferent signals which specify the displacement of the various body segments are centrally monitored and recorded. The first theory is based upon the concept of a proprioceptive inflow (peripheral) model against which, in the absence of exteroceptive information (e.g., auditory, visual, or tactual cues), the central model or efference copy (serving solely as a template or reference mechanism) can be matched. The second position or outflow model is predicated upon the existence of a preprogramed central control mechanism which functions in an open-loop fashion independent of feedback.

Schmidt (1976a) raises three theoretical objections to the inflow model of motor control, the first based upon a problem of communication. Proprioceptive input is encoded in terms of the speed and displacement of limb segments, and the efference or output copy is imprinted in terms of coordinated patterns of muscular contraction (requiring the exertion of precise amounts of force). The inflow model is considered inadequate because it fails to account for the complex recoding processes needed to match the language of the input with that of the output. The second objection is that the inflow model can only correct errors in execution. The inflow model, because it functions by matching the perceived proprioceptive feedback with the temporal and spatial pattern selected by the subject, lacks a mechanism for detecting errors in response selection. If the subject selects an inappropriate response but executes it correctly, there is no way of telling if the environmental goal has been met because there is a perfect match between the feedback and the efference copy, regardless of the consequences of the movement. The third objection to the inflow model is its dependence upon response-produced feedback. Deafferentation studies have revealed that directed movements are still possible even after proprioceptive pathways have been destroyed.

Bossom (1974), for example, reviewed the research on what the transection of the dorsal (sensory) roots of the spinal cord (deafferentation) does to the motor functions of the involved limb segment. He observed that following a postoperative recovery period of suitable duration, experimental animals (monkeys) recovered motor function of the affected limb. These findings apparently contradict the position which contends that the loss of proprioceptive feedback from a limb segment will result in its permanent immobilization, but the restored function did lack the precise refinement which characterizes coordinated movement.

This recovery of function may be attributable to a number of factors. Collateral discharge or central feedback loops which connect different levels of the brain may account for the ability to control movement in the absence of peripheral feedback. It is possible that sensory information from the limb can be conveyed by pathways other than the dorsal root, such as the intact ventral root of the same segment. Another explanation for the recovery of motor function may be the possibility of an increase in the sensitivity of the adjoining intact receptors which exert a compensatory effect. This enables the subject to exert a degree of control over the affected limb. A final factor may result from feedback to muscles which assist the deafferented muscles in the execution of a given movement. Perceived changes in the tension of these helping muscles (synergists) may provide some bases for modulating the force in the affected muscles.

Additional physiological evidence supporting the concept of central motor control is revealed by Taub (1976), who writes that although the movements of deafferented limb segments appear awkward and often lack precision, such movements are nevertheless effective. Since deafferented specimens given special training can learn to perform almost any sequence of movements (with the exception of the most precise) that a normal animal is capable of executing, the author views these findings as strong evidence in support of the motor program concept. Although the principle of a central motor program can account for an organism's capacity to manifest purposive movement in the absence of input from the periphery, such prestructured programs cannot wholly account for the capacity to acquire new skills following deafferentation. In an attempt to reconcile the motor program concept with the plastic nature of learning following deafferentation, Taub proposes two theoretical arguments.

The first hypothesizes the existence of two discrete forms of feedback: topographic, which consists of visual and proprioceptive information concerning the nature and the form of the movement itself; and nontopographic, which pertains only to the environmental consequences or knowledge of results (the reinforcement) of the movement. Topographic or proprioceptive feedback is virtually eliminated by deafferentation. Nontopographic feedback is wholly independent of the information employed in effecting and controlling the movement, and is, therefore, largely unaffected by deafferentation. Although the subject is deprived of the proprioceptive sensations associated with the act of throwing a switch (topographic feedback), the learner is still able to perceive the environmental consequences of the motor activity (e.g., a light going on or a buzzer sounding). Taub theorizes, however, that nontopographic feedback alone cannot result in learning. Hence, a deafferented animal deprived of all topographic feedback (both proprioceptive and visual) must be dependent upon some central control mechanism in order for it to modify its behavior in response to the perceived environmental consequences (nontopographic feedback) of the ongoing activity.

The author's second argument is predicated upon the assumption that learning may be possible in the absence of topographic as well as nontopographic feedback, due to the presence of indelible neural traces or engrams which result from central neurological activity. These traces are believed to constitute a permanent record of a given pattern of activity and serve as a template or reference standard when the initial behavior is to be repeated. Taub contends that these traces, in the complete absence of peripheral feedback, can result solely from central neurological activity.

*Motor Programs.* In view of the theoretical arguments and physiological evidence provided by Jones, Bossom, and Taub, Schmidt (1976a) has proposed an alternative to the inflow or peripheral model, a model which stresses the central role of efferent outflow in the control of movement. This theory is based upon the assumption that the efference copy does not function merely as a template for the evaluation of proprioceptive feedback, but is truly a mechanism capable of serving as the basis for the timing of further efferent signals in the absence of exteroceptive or proprioceptive feedback. Jones (1974a) contends that the outflow model provides an explanation of the ability to perform a movement in the absence of peripheral feedback. Nonetheless, such exteroceptive input is critical during the acquisition of a skill. It appears that the inflow model is representative of the processes related to initial acquisition; the outflow model accounts for the automated response patterns characteristic of high-level skilled performance. In learning to type, for example, the initial phases are characterized by the continual visual monitoring of the symbols to be typed and the position of the fingers on the keyboard. As proficiency is developed, the high response rates characteristic of the skilled typist exceed the individual's capacity to monitor feedback and are therefore indicative of the functioning of a central regulatory mechanism in the control of the movement.

Schmidt (1976b) contends that although the outflow model may constitute a viable explanation for the control of such fine motor activities as typing or the control of eye movements, it cannot account for the adaptations required to compensate for changes in the load or peripheral resistance encountered by the limb segments in the execution of gross motor activities. In the absence of proprioceptive input concerning changes in peripheral resistance, a motor outflow of a predetermined intensity can result in wide fluctuations of motor response. The movement will fall short of the desired goal if the load is increased and will overshoot the goal if the load is decreased. A second objection to the outflow theory is the question of how the efferent commands are monitored. Since the outflow model depends upon some preprogramed reference mechanism for the detection of error, critics of this theory argue that it fails to account adequately for the processes underlying the learning and development of such a mechanism.

Schmidt (1975a) writes that the concept of the motor program or outflow model is largely a default argument since highly speeded movements exceed the learner's capacity to process peripheral feedback. However, Jones (1974a) contends that there is a physiological basis for the outflow model in the circulation of information between the cortex and the cerebellum. This loop system is believed to serve in the discharge of impulses after a fixed delay and thus accounts for the capacity of the central nervous system to preprogram movements and to generate commands in the appropriate temporal sequence. While Jones acknowledges the importance of all modalities of information feedback during the initial acquisition of a motor skill, he argues that in the case of fairly uncomplex, well-practiced skills (e.g., lever positioning), flexible responses are possible in the absence of any form of peripheral feedback. These conclusions are also based upon physiological evidence which indicates that proprioceptive feedback from joint receptors mediates passive movements, and feedback from the muscle spindle is believed to mediate knowledge of force by responding to changes in the load upon a muscle. This function of the muscle spindle is critical in the rapid peripheral regulation of movement at the spinal cord level since such adjustments can be effected in 30 to 50 msc.

Further physiological evidence supporting the central regulation of movement is provided by Brooks (1974), who argues that the programing of movement involves the integrated activity of many parts of the nervous system. Opponents of the central motor program concept argue that such theoretical positions are untenable due to the large number of specific programs which would have to be stored (a separate program for each movement). Brooks contends that any sequence of complicated movements need not necessarily proceed in a stereotyped fashion from beginning to end. He argues that a motor program consists of a series of modular components, each of which is stored in a different part of the nervous system and called upon when needed. These component elements or subroutines range from highly complex patterns of coded neurological information concerning the goals and strategies employed in the execution of the movement to information concerning the force of contraction in the involved muscles. The organization of these constituent elements (subroutines) into a goal-directed behavioral sequence involves the interaction of the peripheral (feedback) and the central (neurological) factors. Each individual element may be used any number of times and in different combinations with other subroutines.

As noted in the preceding discussion, a major objection to the concept of the motor program is that an individual would have to store a specific program for every possible movement. Since, in the English language alone, there are an estimated 100,000 sound patterns or phonemes, and each one would theoretically require a corresponding motor program, the problem of storing the vast number of programs which would be required for all forms of motor activities is formidable. A second objection to the motor program concept is its lack of flexibility. Since no two movements are ever exactly alike—there is always some minor variation in starting position or timing—a specific program would have to be stored for each variation to ensure correct execution in every possible situation. If this should be the case, the already difficult problem of storage is further compounded.

*The Schema Hypothesis.* In light of these objections, Schmidt (1975a) proposes a flexible motor program or schema which accounts for the learner's capacity to generalize a response and thus reduce the number of motor programs which need to be stored. The schema consists of some generalized concept governing a set of objects or events, such as tennis goals and objectives providing the unifying element among the various strokes. While there are many possible variations in the style of each stroke, particularly in the serve, each variant is nevertheless recognizable in terms of general properties associated with the intended purpose of the stroke (the goal of the movement). Rumelhart (1977) describes a schema as a hypothetical system which accounts for an individual's capacity to abstract a set of observed features from a given cue in the input. This cue may be verbal in nature, entailing either a letter or a word, or it may consist of some form of sensory stimulus such as light, sound, or proprioceptive feedback. In the past, learning theorists have traditionally confined their research to the study of such molecular behaviors as the conditioned reflex. The schema offers a hypothesis designed to account for very complex, high-order learning (molar behavior).

Perhaps one of the greatest attractions of the schema hypothesis is its high degree of plasticity. It freely allows the learner to condense or elaborate the basic elements contained in the information input. This plasticity is the result of the bi-directionality of the schema hypothesis; it can function either from the top down or from the bottom up. In the latter case, lower-level hypotheses (reflexes, in the case of motor learning) are combined into higher-order behaviors or subroutines which are themselves combined into still more complex, purposive patterns of goal-directed movement.

In the case of verbal learning, for example, the presence of a particular letter may suggest a variety of words in which that letter can be used. A person watching a child playing with alphabet blocks looks at the letter "C" and thinks briefly about his car parked outside. In a motor learning situation, the presence of a piece of gymnasium apparatus or sports equipment can serve as a stimulus for initiating a complex behavioral adaptation associated with the execution of a particular sports activity, such as a routine on the parallel bars or the swing of a tennis racket or golf club. Conversely, the schema can also operate from the top down in that higher-level hypotheses concerning goals and objectives will result in the selection of the appropriate lower-level responses required to achieve these goals. A golfer whose goal it is to hit the ball off the tee ultimately attains this end by employing the necessary precise, specific, neuromuscular responses.

It must be remembered, however, that although the schema theory provides a promising avenue of research concerning the role of information processing in motor learning, it is still in its infancy and remains highly speculative in nature. It will be some time before researchers in the area are able to generate the experimental evidence and the theoretical sophistication needed to determine its true value. Schmidt (1976b), a leading proponent of the application of the schema theory to motor learning, argues that the schema is actually an abstraction of a set of stimuli and is dependent upon four factors: the initial conditions, the response specifications for the motor program, the sensory consequences (feedback) of the response produced, and the outcome of the movement (environmental consequences).

The initial conditions are perceived in terms of both internal and environmental cues. Proprioceptive feedback provides information concerning the position of the body in space and the acceleration and displacement (speed and position) of the limb segments. Exteroceptive information concerning the state of the environment is conveyed through auditory and visual feedback. Both the proprioceptive and exteroceptive information are utilized in the formulation of the movement strategy and are then stored in memory for future reference.

The matter of response specification refers to the constraints placed upon the general program or schema in the execution of a particular movement. Although the motor program for the tennis serve may be endowed with the capacity for eliciting a number of possible responses, a particular game situation may call for a highly specific response. Such a response is determined by precise variations in the intensity and duration of muscular force, ultimately resulting in a unique pattern of movement. Following the execution of the skill, information pertaining to the movement pattern is stored along with other response-produced feedback information and serves as a precise record of the movement produced.

The sensory consequences of a movement consist of an exact copy of the afferent information provided by the proprioceptive and the exteroceptive response-produced information feedback. This information is stored in memory and can be readily retrieved when the movement is repeated.

The response outcome is determined by the environmental consequences of a motor act and is a function of the degree of discrepancy between the response desired (e.g., hitting a baseball) and the actual response attained (missing because the swing was too late). Information pertaining to the response outcome is stored following the movement and can consist of knowledge of results in the form of verbal correction by a teacher or coach, or subjective reinforcement by the learner who is aware of the consequences of the movement in the absence of KR (e.g., holding a handstand or scoring a basket). The KR may consist of a quantitatively precise definition of error (such as "three degrees too far to the left") or may entail some qualitative statement (such as "too slow" or "too fast"); the subjective reinforcement is, in contrast, wholly dependent upon the perceived consequences of the response as conveyed through exteroceptive information feedback.

The stored information pertaining to the initial conditions, response specifications, sensory consequences, and response outcomes can be recalled and combined in varying proportions. The flexibility inherent in the resultant response pattern becomes the basis of the motor schema by providing a regulatory function that is both comprehensive and adaptable to a variety of situations. Schmidt (1976b) proposes a two-stage model of the motor response schema. The first stage consists of the recall schema which is instrumental both in the execution of movement and in the correction of movement errors. The second stage consists of the recognition schema which evaluates response-produced feedback and generates error information.

At this point, the respective roles of recall and recognition (concepts initiated within the study of verbal retention) should be clarified. Adams (1971) contends that recall is analogous to the memory trace and is therefore critical to the selection and initiation of a movement. In contrast, recognition corresponds to the perceptual trace and is central to the regulation and control of the ongoing movement. Wallace and McGhee (1979) write that recognition memory is developed as a consequence of the learner's association of KR with the feedback from the various sensory modalities. It is through this contiguous association that the learner is able to develop an internalized model (the recognition memory or perceptual trace) for evaluating performance-generated feedback in the absence of KR. Recall memory is strengthened through the association of the efferent commands (response specifications) with the KR. Over a period of time the learner develops an internalized standard of movement production (the recall memory or the memory trace), and the required response specifications can be initiated in the absence of KR. Sensory feedback is believed to be critical only to the formation of recognition memory; response specifications are confined to the formation of recall memory; KR is central to the formation of both memory states.

The respective functions of the recall schema and the recognition schema are dependent upon different sources of information. The recall schema is based upon the relationships established among the initial conditions, the response specifications and the actual response outcome. These relationships are strengthened through practice and continually refined through each succeeding trial. When the ordered pattern of interaction among these three constituent elements has been well established, the recall schema can be employed in the execution of a novel response even though only the initial conditions and desired outcomes are known. The organizational rules governing the schema will supply the necessary response specifications for the execution of the novel task. An individual who can hit a tennis ball landing to his right side is capable of adapting that response to play a ball landing to his left.

The recognition schema operates in a similar fashion, and is concerned with the variables pertaining to initial conditions, sensory consequences, and actual outcomes (KR). The strength of the recognition schema is a function of the degree of association between the sensory consequences (the exteroceptive and proprioceptive feedback) and the actual outcome. After these responses have been paired a number of times during the course of practice, the learner is able to predict the expected sensory consequences, provided the desired response has been specified. Schmidt (1976b) argues that the recognition schema constitutes the basis for the learning of rapid movements in the absence of KR since the actual sensory consequences can be compared with the expected sensory consequences. Any resultant discrepancy between these two values will indicate that an error has been made in the execution of the movement and will provide the subject with information about the accuracy of his response, even in the absence of KR.

The concept of a flexible motor program or schema is given further support by Powell, Katzko, and Royce (1978), who argue that neither traditional motor program theories nor simple closed-loop feedback models can provide an adequate explanation of the control processes involved in the regulation of complex movement. Since skilled movement patterns are rarely identical (e.g., every ball thrown by a pitcher will behave in a manner that is slightly different from every other pitch), the central control processes governing the performance of such complex activities must be flexible and capable of rapid adaptations. Further, skilled performance is possible even in the absence of feedback or knowledge of results, and the rapid response times associated with the execution of certain motor skills often exceeds the maximal rate with which an individual can process information feedback.

A final argument in favor of an open-loop, flexible program concept of motor control is based upon the factor of motor equivalence, or equifinality. This principle is regarded by the authors as further evidence of the flexible nature of motor control processes since an individual is able to carry out a variety of motor acts by employing body segments other than those involved in the initial acquisition of the task. The application of this principle is most evident in rehabilitation programs for the handicapped in which an individual may be taught to write by holding a pen with the teeth while forming the letters with movements of the head, or may learn to use the legs and feet to execute a task previously relegated to the hands and arms.

Powell et al. (1978) hypothesize a multi-stage flexible motor program which integrates cognitive decision processes, motor memory, neurological control mechanisms, and individual difference factors. This flexible program or schema accounts for an individual's capacity to process large amounts of highly complex information in a rapid and efficient manner. For example, the first component of a schema for learning to write would consist of a control mechanism governing the formation of a series of basic strokes, such as lines, dots, and circles; the second stage would involve a set of rules or principles for combining the strokes into letters; the third stage would entail a still more highly ordered set of rules for combining the letters into words. The final stage of such a flexible program would involve the most complex level of organization, the combination of words into phrases and sentences. Although the example pertains to the acquisition of a fine motor activity, the same rules and principles govern the acquisition of gross motor skills since it is only through practice and repetition that basic elements of a task are combined into more complex behavioral units or "chunks." Paradoxically, as the length and complexity of these behavioral chunks or subroutines increases, the role of conscious intervention in their regulation and control diminishes. As learning proceeds, the integration of behavior becomes an increasingly automated function.

Combining basic elements of behavior into more complex patterns (chunking) results in the creation of higher-order rules which govern the newly formed higher-order behavior units or components. Powell et al. contend that increasing the length and complexity of the behavioral unit through the combination and interaction of the more basic behavioral elements constitutes the principal factor underlying the increased degree of automatic control. Apparently, the greater the tendency of the learner to process large amounts of complexly patterned information, the more automatic the functioning of the neurological mechanisms which process this information. A young child who is just learning to play the piano requires far more conscious effort to "pick out" the notes of a simple melody than does an accomplished virtuoso performing a highly difficult work. The acquisition of skill apparently entails the capacity for organizing and patterning individual movements into purposive, goal-directed activities; the greater the proficiency of the learner, the more quickly and efficiently this end is accomplished. Although a complex movement pattern is consciously initiated (since there is an objective or goal to be accomplished, ideational activity is involved), its regulation and control are carried on at subconscious levels. The higher the level of proficiency, the greater the degree of automation in the regulation of a given movement.

*Other Information-Processing Models.* Although the schema theory provides a promising albeit speculative approach to the mechanisms which underlie the acquisition and control of complex, goal-directed movement patterns, it is only one of a number of theoretical positions which have been developed. Smith (1970) argues that learning and memory are time-spanning processes which are determined by spatial and temporal factors inherent in information feedback. He contends that learning occurs most efficiently when the pattern of response persists as a perceived, operational, sensory feedback effect of movement (a motor memory trace), which creates a spanned temporal record of past response. The more complete this persisting spatial feedback pattern, the more rapid and efficient the learning and the more complete the memory record. However, the memory trace is more than a mere record of past movement and perception since it functions as a dynamic, time-spanning process in the form of a feedforward control system which projects movement into the future. It is through this projection mechanism that a learner is believed to anticipate a given situation or respond to a novel one (an outfielder getting the jump on the ball or a skier traversing a new trail).

Learning and memory function, in effect, as interdependent feedback and feedforward mechanisms which integrate movements over particular spans of space and time. Such temporal and spatial integrative processes account for the learner's capacity to predict the course of future movements and to project the path of moving objects. Smith contends that the motor memory constitutes a predictive and anticipatory feedforward control process which develops as a direct consequence of learning. The information feedback emanating from the ongoing activity is stored by the learner and ultimately serves in the selection and guidance of future response patterns.

Adams (1977) writes that feedback concerning the temporal and spatial patterning of a motor skill is generated by peripheral receptors in the involved limb segments. Through practice reinforced by knowledge of results, this information is ultimately transformed and encoded in the form of a perceptual trace which serves as a model or template for the smooth and automatic execution of the skill following its initial acquisition. The activity of the somatosensory cortex (the area of the brain in which peripheral feedback is centrally recorded) is an accurate linear approximation of the firing patterns of the peripheral receptors. The building of a perceptual trace for the retention and execution of rapid, extrinsically-paced movements is dependent upon a further transformation of this afferent feedback which is nonlinear in nature. Unfortunately, the nature of these nonlinear transformations which underlie the cortical association processes for the analysis and inter-pretation of afferent input are as yet unknown.

Sommerhoff (1974) writes that learning is dependent upon the interaction of neural networks which register relationships between environmental (stimulus) and movement variables. He contends that through the process of directive correlation, relationships are established which govern the control of these variables and enable the learner to develop expectations concerning the degree to which stimuli will vary in response to certain movements. An experienced hitter knows that by contacting the ball with the bat at a particular point in its flight, the course of the ball will be radically altered. Once such relationships have been established, the learner can pursue a goal-directed activity even if there is a momentary disruption in the flow of information feedback, such as the loss of visual input when blinking the eyes. A skilled performer, however, is not affected by such temporary disruptions in feedback.

Sommerhoff defines directive correlation as a process by which an organism, through the continual modification of its behavior, can achieve some environmental goal. Information (feedback) concerning the environmental conditions is centrally processed by the organism and, as a result, responses are effected which are linked or correlated to these prevailing conditions. (These conditions, in turn, determine the response elicited.) Sommerhoff defined three types of directive correla-tion : 1) immediate, as in the case of a skilled performer in the martial arts responding to an attack; 2) long-term, which refers to responses which have been acquired and refined over many years of practice, as in a professional tennis player's performance; and 3) biological, which refers to the changes in the nervous system which have evolved over many thousands of years and which enable humans to elicit many highly complex levels of goal-directed activity. The capacity for language and abstract reasoning constitutes a prime example of biological adaptations which have resulted in profound behavioral modifications.

Sommerhoff acknowledges the concept of the schema but views its function as limited to serving merely as a template or internal model which facilitates the processing of information. Although the schema can provide a mechanism which enables the learner to anticipate or predict the future course of a movement, thus allowing him to function in the absence of information feedback for limited periods of time (open-loop behavior), two highly similar stimulus situations can result in the schema's automatic selection of an erroneous response. Although the schema concept can provide a valuable adjunct to understanding the mechanisms of motor control, it apparently cannot, in and of itself, satisfactorily account for the processes which underlie the capacity to discriminate precisely between similar stimuli and effect an appropriate response. The schema, in essence, may well be only one of many factors operating in the control of movement.

Glencross (1977) writes that although the execution of precise patterns of highly speeded movements apparently exceeds the learner's capacity to process the feedback information derived from the continual monitoring of the ongoing activity, any blockage or distortion of such information ultimately results in a decrease in proficiency. These findings imply that for any central control process (motor program) to be fully effective, it must be integrated at some point with peripheral sensory information. The major problems pertain to how the integration occurs and to the precise way in which the feedback is used to facilitate the ongoing central organization. Glencross proposes a two-stage model of motor control which involves an executive component, dependent upon information feedback, and a motor program component, which functions in an open-loop fashion. The motor program, once it has been initiated, will run its full course without any further sensory or central intervention, but the executive program continually monitors the ongoing response. This monitoring is particularly intensive during the early stages of skill acquisition. As competence is acquired, the basic units of the activity (the unitary subroutines or bits) are combined into more complex and predictable (redundant) sequences of action. These behavior sequences are temporarily integrated by the executive program which, as a result, is then able to monitor organized patterns of movement rather than individual movements.

The processing of feedback information derived from complex, integrated movement patterns requires between 300 and 500 msc.; the processing time for decisions and responses concerning discrete stimuli runs from about 150 to 200 msc. These time lags are far too long to account for the rapid organizational processes involved in regulating complex sequences of motor activity and those less complex processes involved in error correction and the formation of strategies for response modification. In the light of this problem, Glencross proposes a series of theoretical explanations which attempt to account for an individual's capacity to process information feedback at considerably higher rates.

The first of these pertains to the predictability or redundancy of the feedback signal itself. When a skill is intensively practiced, the resultant feedback or error signal becomes increasingly predictable, thus reducing the need for its continual routine analysis by the lower motor regulatory centers. Glencross theorizes that when feedback is highly redundant, as in the case of a well-learned skill, a direct communication link is established between the error signal and the motor program. It is estimated that the formation of such a direct pathway can reduce response time to 80 msc.

The labeling or coding of feedback signals in terms of varying their quantitative temporal and spatial features or their gain or amplification constitutes a second factor believed to facilitate the central processing of information feedback. Glencross writes that there is evidence to indicate that signal modifications involving only gain or amplification can be produced very rapidly and can result in general timing adjustments as well as the correction of directional errors. It is argued that specifically labeled patterns of alternative movements are stored in memory and can be immediately triggered by the appropriately coded pattern of information feedback. For example, for every ongoing movement there is a stored program for an equal but opposite movement which can be elicited by the appropriately coded pattern of feedback and which will exert a rapid compensatory effect upon the ongoing activity.

The concept of central matching of feedback and feedforward constitutes the third theoretical position concerning the basis of rapid error corrections and response modifications. It is similar to the outflow model proposed by Jones: the output from the motor program is continually monitored by a central regulatory mechanism which is itself programed by peripheral feedback. This center is believed to possess the capacity to effect adjustments in the execution of the motor program within 50 msc. and to function as part of the executive system. Glencross writes that these central regulatory mechanisms, in addition to decreasing response time, provide flexibility since their function enables one motor program to achieve a variety of related responses. This factor is of practical importance, for it implies that it is not necessary to postulate a different motor program for each separate skilled movement. Glencross writes, in conclusion, that an understanding of the basis of motor control is dependent upon further knowledge concerning the integration of central and peripheral processes. Particular attention needs to be given to the question of how an executive system is capable of processing a variety of feedback signals and to the ways in which this information can be used to modify the motor program that ultimately determines the organization of the ongoing skilled response.

Schmidt (1980) writes that both peripheral feedback and central programing are critical factors in the regulation and control of movement, and that the relative importance of each varies with the parameters of the criterion task. Very rapid movements are more likely to fall under the control of preprogramed central processes, while slow movements lend themselves to regulation through the monitoring of peripheral feedback. Tasks which require high levels of selective attention (such as team sport skills) are more likely to fall under preprogramed central control since the active processing of information feedback will place additional demands upon the learner's attentional capacity. The greater the degree of automation with which a skill is executed, the greater the reliance upon central programing. Schmidt argues that the acquisition of motor skills entails central as well as peripheral mechanisms which function in synergy and provide the learner with a degree of flexibility which enables him or her to process different types of information under a wide range of environmental circumstances. Schmidt's contention concerning the respective importance of central and peripheral mechanisms in motor learning is substantiated by Glencross and Gould (1979), who write that the fundamental issues in the control of movement pertain to 1) which details of the response can be prepared in advance, and 2) the role of feedback mechanisms during the course of its execution.

The various information-processing models discussed in this chapter are predicated upon the premise that motor learning is a process dependent upon the temporal and spatial integration of muscular responses. Such integration may result from the influence of a central motor program or the monitoring of peripheral information feedback. Controversy exists over which of these mechanisms is the most critical factor in motor learning. Current research concerning the structure and function of the nervous system tends to indicate that the learning of complex, goal-directed motor skills is most probably dependent upon the interaction of both mechanisms. Proficiency is ultimately dependent upon the learner's capacity to combine individual movements into complex, goal-directed patterns through the temporal and spatial integration of sensory feedback.

Learning involves two apparently opposing processes which actually function in synergy: the reduction and simplification of information, and its structuring and synthesis. The first function of learning pertains to the reduction of uncertainty initially associated with the acquisition of a novel skill. The second phase concerns the synthesis of basic responses into an ordered, purposive sequence of behavior. The acquisition of complex motor skills is in effect a function of the learner's capacity to organize a series of specific responses into a unified, purposive pattern of behavior. Prior to acquisition, the learner is confronted with a high degree of uncertainty (the total of the uncertainty associated with each separate response). As proficiency develops, the individual responses are combined into a unified, purposive behavioral pattern, and there is a corresponding reduction in the uncertainty that the learner must resolve. As the organization of the response pattern increases, the uncertainty initially associated with the component elements of that pattern decreases.

It is evident that the acquisition and performance of purposive, complex, goal-directed motor skills are dependent upon central and peripheral processes which enable the learner to interact dynamically with the environment. Identifying and clarifying the specific functional interrelationships among these information-processing mechanisms becomes the major challenge to theoretical and experimental research in motor learning. Once the functional basis of motor activity is understood, it will be possible to better predict and control the interactions among such factors as the nature and conditions of practice, the individual differences of the learner, and the taxonomical characteristics of the criterion task. It is hoped that scientific fact will ultimately supplant the trial-and-error methods currently employed in the teaching of motor skills. The practical consequences of such a scientifically oriented approach which matches the requirements of the task to the capacities of the learner will be reflected in a greater number of individuals realizing productive and rewarding experiences in the learning of motor tasks.

*References*

Adams, J.A. "A Closed-Loop Theory of Motor Learning." *Journal of Motor Behavior, 3* (1971), 111–149.

_____. "Feedback Theory of How Joint Receptors Regulate the Timing and Positioning of a Limb." *Psychological Review, 84* (1977), 504–523.

_____ and S. Dijkstra. "Short-Term Memory for Motor Responses." *Journal of Experimental Psychology, 71* (1966), 314–318.

Bossom, J. "Movement Without Proprioception." *Brain Research, 71* (1974), 285–296.

Broadbent, D.E. "Recent Analyses of Short-Term Memory." *In* K.H. Pribram and D.E. Broadbent (eds.), *Biology of Memory*. New York: Academic Press, 1970.

Brooks, V.B. "Some Examples of Programed Limb Movements." *Brain Research, 71* (1974), 297–308.

Gentile, A.M. and J. Nacson. "Organizational Processes in Motor Control." *In* J. Keogh and R.S. Hutton (eds.), *Exercise and Sport Science Reviews.* Santa Barbara, Cal.: Journal Publishing Affiliates, 1976.

Glencross, D.J. "Control of Skilled Movements." *Psychological Bulletin, 84* (1977), 14–29.

―――― and J.M. Gould. "The Planning of Precision Movements." *Journal of Motor Behavior, 11* (1979), 1–9.

Henry, F.M. "Variable and Constant Performance Errors Within a Group of Individuals." *Journal of Motor Behavior, 6* (1974), 149–154.

Jones, B. "Is Proprioception Important for Skilled Performance?" *Journal of Motor Behavior, 6* (1974a), 33–45.

――――. "Role of Central Monitoring of Efference in Short-Term Memory for Movements." *Journal of Experimental Psychology, 102* (1974b), 37–43.

Laabs, J.G. "A Note Concerning the Effect of Kinesthetic Memory Load on the Retention of Movement End-Location." *Journal of Motor Behavior, 8* (1976), 313–316.

Marteniuk, R.G. "Cognitive Information Processes in Motor Short-Term Memory and Movement Production." *In* G.E. Stelmach (ed.), *Motor Control Issues and Trends.* New York: Academic Press, 1976.

Melton, A.W. "Short- and Long-Term Postperceptual Memory: Dichotomy or Continuum?" *In* K.H. Pribram and D.E. Broadbent (eds.), *Biology of Memory,* New York: Academic Press, 1970.

Newell, K.M. "Knowledge of Results and Motor Learning." *In* J. Keogh and R.S. Hutton (eds.), *Exercise and Sport Science Reviews.* Santa Barbara, Cal.: Journal Publishing Affiliates, 1976a.

――――. "Motor Learning Without Knowledge of Results Through the Development of a Response Recognition Mechanism." *Journal of Motor Behavior, 8* (1976b), 209–217.

Powell, A., M. Katzko, and K.R. Royce. "A Multifactor-Systems Theory of the Structure and Dynamics of Motor Functions." *Journal of Motor Behavior, 10* (1978), 191–210.

Roy, E.A. "Measuring Change in Motor Memory." *Journal of Motor Behavior, 8* (1976), 283–287.

Rumelhart, D. *Introduction to Human Information Processing.* New York: John Wiley, 1977.

Schendel, J.D. and K.M. Newell. "On Processing the Information from Knowledge of Results." *Journal of Motor Behavior, 8* (1976), 251–255.

Schmidt, R.A. "A Schema Theory of Discrete Motor Skill Learning." *Psychological Review, 82* (1975a), 251–255.

_____. *Motor Skills.* New York: Harper and Row, 1975b.

_____. "Control Processes in Motor Skills." *In* J. Keogh and R.S. Hutton (eds.), *Exercise and Sport Science Reviews.* Santa Barbara, Cal.: Journal Publishing Affiliates, 1976a.

_____. "The Schema As a Solution to Some Persistent Problems in Motor Learning Theory." *In* G.E. Stelmach (ed.), *Motor Control Issues and Trends,* New York: Academic Press, 1976b.

_____. "Past and Future Issues in Motor Programing." *Research Quarterly for Exercise and Sport, 51* (1980), 122–140.

Smith, K.U. and G. "Feedback Mechanism of Athletic Skill." *In* L.E. Smith (ed.), *Psychology of Motor Learning.* Chicago: The Athletic Institute, 1970.

Sommerhoff, G. *Logic of the Living Brain.* New York: John Wiley, 1974.

Stelmach, G.E., J.S. Kelso, and P.D. McCullagh. "Preselection and Response Biasing in Short-Term Motor Memory." *Memory and Cognition, 4* (1976), 62–66.

_____ and M. Wilson. "Kinesthetic Retention, Movement Extent, and Information Processing." *Journal of Experimental Psychology, 85* (1970), 425–430.

Taub, E. "Movement in Nonhuman Primates Deprived of Somatosensory Feedback." *In* J. Keogh and R.S. Hutton (eds.), *Exercise and Sport Science Reviews.* Santa Barbara, Cal.: Journal Publishing Affiliates, 1976.

Tulving, E. "Short- and Long-Term Memory: Different Retrieval Mechanisms." *In* K.H. Pribram and D.E. Broadbent (eds.), *Biology of Memory.* New York: Academic Press, 1970.

Wallace, S.A. and R.C. McGhee. "The Independence of Recall and Recognition in Motor Learning." *Journal of Motor Behavior, 11* (1979), 141–151.

# Index